Discussions in Patient Management

GRAVES' DISEASE

By

ALAN E. LEWIS, M.D.
Associate Professor of Medicine
Hahnemann Medical College and Hospital
Philadelphia, Pennsylvania

with chapters by:

Norman G. Schneeberg, M.D.
Professor of Medicine

Thomas Moshang, M.D.
Associate Professor of Pediatrics

Saul Weinstein, M.D.
Assistant Professor of Surgery

Hahnemann Medical College and Hospital
Philadelphia, Pennsylvania

 Medical Examination Publishing Co., Inc.
an Excerpta Medica company

Garden City, New York

Copyright © 1980 by
MEDICAL EXAMINATION PUBLISHING CO., INC.
an Excerpta Medica company

Library of Congress Card Number
80-15624

ISBN 0-87488-870-0

July, 1980

All rights reserved. No part of this
publication may be reproduced in any
form or by any means, electronic or
mechanical, including photocopy,
without permission in writing from
the publisher.

Printed in the United States of America

SIMULTANEOUSLY PUBLISHED IN:

Europe : HANS HUBER PUBLISHERS
Bern, Switzerland

Preface

Graves' Disease, Discussions in Patient Management was written to present the concepts of treating hyperthyroidism to any physician interested in handling this disease. The general discussion in each chapter should lead the reader to the application of a specific aspect of therapy to each individual patient. The case histories have been selected to illustrate these points of therapy as well as to answer questions frequently asked about these principles. To permit a comprehensive view of the subject, the text has been divided into general discussions of topics such as drug therapy and treatments of quite specific matters such as the treatment of hyperthyroidism in childhood. This permits the illustration of general principles, as well as potential modifications of these principles that may be necessary. The author hopes that the explanations will allow for evaluation of future developments in therapy. The references are as complete as possible for a text of this size. These citations should permit the reader to pursue his own examination of the subject.

Several acknowledgements are in order. Thanks are extended to Dr. Norman Schneeberg and to Dr. Joseph Gambescia for comments that helped improve several chapters. Needless to say, the final version remains that of the author. It is impossible to express the appreciation due my family, particularly my wife Sandra, whose continual encouragement and tolerance made completion of this project possible.

Main premise

Stone should never have stopped my successful therapy. There was no medical reason to do so. In addition I begged him to restore it because I didn't feel well. He talked me out of that

Contents

Handwritten annotations:
Similarly, takes 6-8 weeks for medication to be out of system. Dr. Stone should have had me return for later tests & especially for T3 which was never done.

But most important therapy should not have been stopped.

I	DIAGNOSIS OF HYPERTHYROIDISM . . . . by Norman G. Schneeberg, M.D.	1
II	TREATMENT OF HYPERTHYROIDISM: GENERAL CONSIDERATIONS	18
III	DRUG THERAPY OF HYPERTHYROIDISM . . . . . Part One: Thioamides . . . . Part Two: Drugs Other Than Thioamides	23 24 44
IV	SURGERY AND HYPERTHYROIDISM . . . . Appendix: Technique of Surgery . . . . by Saul Weinstein, M.D.	53 67
V	RADIOIODINE	72
VI	HYPERTHYROIDISM IN CHILDHOOD . . . . by Thomas Moshang, M.D.	91
VII	SPECIAL PROBLEMS IN THE TREATMENT OF HYPERTHYROIDISM . . . . Hyperthyroidism in Pregnancy . . . . Thyroid Storm . . . . Ophthalmopathy . . . . Unusual Forms of Hyperthyroidism . . . . Apathetic Hyperthyroidism	100 101 105 110 113 115
	INDEX	122

notice

The editor(s) and/or author(s) and the publisher of this book have made every effort to ensure that all therapeutic modalities that are recommended are in accordance with accepted standards at the time of publication.

The drugs specified within this book may not have specific approval by the Food and Drug Administration in regard to the indications and dosages that are recommended by the editor(s) and/or author(s). The manufacturer's package insert is the best source of current prescribing information.

CHAPTER I

DIAGNOSIS OF HYPERTHYROIDISM

Norman G. Schneeberg, M.D.

Body metabolism is maintained in part by an adequate milieu of circulating thyroid hormones (TH), thyroxine (T4) and triiodothyronine (T3). An excessive concentration of TH and their impact upon body cells produce the clinical manifestations of hyperthyroidism. Though the most prevalent variety of hyperthyroidism is Graves' Disease, proper recognition of other causes, outlined in Table I.1, is essential for accurate diagnosis and successful therapy.

GRAVES' DISEASE

Graves' Disease is currently viewed as an autoimmune disorder provoked by the elaboration of either a thyroid-stimulating immunoglobulin or a spectrum of closely related immunoglobulins responsible for goiter, thyroid hypersecretion, opthalmopathy and sometimes dermopathy, acropachy, splenomegaly, lymphadenopathy and thymic hyperplasia. The triad of hyperthyroidism, goiter, and opthalmopathy usually co-exist but occasionally one or two of these manifestations precede the others, as in Euthyroid Graves' Disease.

2/ Diagnosis of Hyperthyroidism

TABLE I.1

A CLASSIFICATION OF HYPERTHYROIDISM

1. Graves' Disease (toxic diffuse goiter)
   a) Hyperthyroidism, diffuse goiter, ophthalmopathy
   b) Euthyroid Graves' Disease
   c) T3-thyrotoxicosis*

2. Plummer's Disease (toxic nodular goiter)
   a) Toxic adenomatous goiter
   b) Hyperthyroidism with nodular goiter

3. Transient "Hyperthyroidism" - subacute thyroiditis, post- 131-I therapy, neo-natal (LATS)

4. Thyroid carcinoma (follicular)

5. Thyrotrophin (TSH) induced
   a) with pituitary tumor
   b) without pituitary tumor
   c) ectopic: choriocarcinoma, mole, teratocarcinoma, bronchiogenic carcinoma (probably HCG)

6. Struma ovarii

7. Jodbasedow (iodide-induced)

8. Thyrotoxicosis factitia and medicamentosa

9. Hashimoto's Chronic Thyroiditis with hyperthyroidism ("Hashitoxicosis")

---

* also in toxic nodular goiter

HYPERTHYROIDISM

Symptoms include nervousness, restlessness, tremors, sweating, heat intolerance, cold preference, weight loss despite an increased caloric intake, fatigue, weakness and palpitations. Less frequent complaints include bulging eyes, irritation of eyelids and/or lacrimation, eye fatigue, diplopia, hyperdefecation, pruritus, swelling of legs and dyspnea. Important physical signs are goiter, thyroid bruit, tachycardia, occasionally atrial fibrillation, widened pulse pressure, fine digital tremor, moist, satin-smooth skin, and hyperkinesis. Occasionally there is myopathy, localized myxedema, onycholysis or acropachy. The presence or absence of certain clinical phenomena has been employed by Crooks et al[1] to derive a "clinical index" which may be of diagnostic value.

SYMPTOMS

	PRESENT	ABSENT
Dyspnea on effort	+1	--
Palpitations	+2	--
Tiredness	+2	--
Preference for heat	--	-5
Preference for cold	+5	--
Sweating	+3	--
Nervousness	+2	--
Appetite increased	+3	--
Appetite decreased	--	-3
Weight decreased	+3	--
Weight increased	--	-3

SIGNS

	PRESENT	ABSENT
Palpable thyroid	+3	-3
Thyroid bruit	+2	-2
Exophthalmos	+2	--
Lid retraction	+2	--
Lid lag	+1	--
Hyperkinesis	+4	-2
Digital tremor	+1	--
Hands - hot	+2	-2
Hands - moist	+1	-1
Atrial fibrillation	+4	--

(cont'd.)

4/ Diagnosis of Hyperthyroidism

(cont'd.)

		PRESENT	ABSENT
	80	--	-3
Casual pulse rate	80-90	0	--
	90	+3	--

SCORE

Euthyroid	+11
Hyperthyroid	+19
Equivocal	+11 to +19

In the elderly and during pregnancy symptoms and signs may be considerably blunted. Occasionally an apathetic form of hyperthyroidism is encountered particularly in older patients. Thus the clinical picture of hyperthyroidism may encompass a spectrum ranging from almost complete absence of symptoms to the most extreme variety of thyrotoxicosis, namely crisis. The physical signs may exhibit a similar range, i.e., from so-called "masked thyrotoxicosis" to florid hyperthyroidism. Rarely the disease may be first appreciated when laboratory tests reveal elevations of circulating TH and only after careful probing one can elicit significant symptoms from the patient. End-organ tissue sensitivity to thyroid hormones may show considerable variation resulting in atypical clinical responses. Thus a jogger's normal heart rate of 50/min. may rise to only 65 to 70 when thyrotoxic. The diagnosis of hyperthyroidism becomes difficult when clinical manifestations are muted or when manifestations related to one body system overshadow other manifestations.

Some atypical manifestations or presentations of hyperthyroidism are:

1. Apathy, depression, psychosis
2. Thyrotoxic myopathy
3. Encephalopathy, epilepsy
4. GI manifestations - chronic diarrhea, abdominal pain simulating pepetic ulcer, vomiting
5. Peripheral edema
6. Pruritus
7. Hypercalcemia
8. Periodic paralysis
9. Myasthenia Gravis
10. Congestive Heart Failure

Opthalmopathy is found in most patients with Graves' Disease. Two varieties are recognized:

1. Non-infiltrative (mild) form that consists of stare, infrequent blinking and lid-lag. Occasionally mild extraocular muscle weakness may occur though this is usually a manifestation of the more severe variety described below. Non-infiltrative ophthalmopathy is an expression of the impact of excessive amounts of circulating TH and is found in all varieties of hyperthyroidism. The upper eyelids are retracted from increased sympathetic tone of Muller's superior palpebral muscle, a direct consequence of increased T4 and T3. Successful treatment of hyperthyroidism usually relieves the retraction completely unless it has been of very long duration when fibrosis and permanent retraction of the upper eyelids can occur.

2. Infiltrative ophthalmopathy (severe, progressive) is caused by extraocular muscle hypertrophy and degeneration together with an increase in retro-orbital fluid, fat, mucopolysaccharides and fibrous tissue. There is exophthalmos, periorbital and eyelid edema, extraocular muscle weakness often resulting in diploplia, ophalmoplegia, conjunctival and scleral injection and edema (chemosis). The patient may experience lacrimation, irritation and pain, photophobia, diplopia and blurred vision. Infiltration of Muller's muscle may promote permanent retraction due to fibrotic shortening. Similar fibrosis of extraocular muscles with muscle shortening can result in fixed strabismus. In severe infiltrative ophthalmopathy, particularly with lagophthalmos, exposure keratitis and corneal ulceration can threaten vision. Occasionally there may be decreased visual acuity, papilledema, scotomata and visual field impairment.

It should be emphasized that the manifestations of ophthalmopathy often bear no relationship to the severity of hyperthyroidism. Some extremely toxic patients exhibit the non-infiltrative form, and some of the mildest forms of hyperthyroidism may be associated with severe progressive (malignant) ophthalmopathy. Non-infiltrative forms can progress to the infiltrative variety.

6/ Diagnosis of Hyperthyroidism

The previously mentioned classification of the eye change of hyperthyroidism may be overly simplified since it is based on clinical judgement alone. Recent evidence[2] using ultrasonography of the orbit of patients with Graves' Disease showed that orbital involvement was almost universal and consisted principally of enlargement of the extraocular muscles. Thus the classification "non-infiltrative ophthalmopathy" may be outmoded.

A more detailed and informative classification of Graves' ophthalmopathy was proposed in 1969.[3] An abridged form is as follows:

Class	
0	No signs or symptoms
1	Only signs, no symptoms (signs limited to upper lid retraction and stare with or without lig lag and proptosis).
2	Soft tissue involvement (symptoms and signs)
3	Proptosis
4	Extraocular muscle involvement
5	Corneal involvement
6	Sight loss (optic nerve involvement)

The ophthalmic changes of Graves' Disease cannot always be as clearly defined; many patients show a mixed picture suggesting both the non-infiltrative and infiltrative form. It is very likely that a single basic etiologic process is responsible for all the eye changes of Graves' Disease. The most recent classification of these eye changes has been proposed by the American Thyroid Association.[4]

TOXIC ADENOMATOUS GOITER (TAG)

This form of hyperthyroidism is caused by an autonomously hyperfunctioning thyroid adenoma (or adenomata) and is distinct from Graves' Disease. The adenoma (or adenomata) is usually easily palpable; small nodules rarely induce thyrotoxicosis. In the USA only 5-10% of hyperthyroid patients are TAG though in other parts of the world 1/4 to 1/3 of all cases are TAG. TAG is a true thyroid disorder and is unrelated to autoimmune mechanisms. Features distinctive from Graves' Disease are shown in Table I.2. Cardiovascular manifestations, especially in the elderly, can obscure other signs of thyrotoxicosis and the term "masked thyrotoxicosis" is often employed in such instances. Paroxysmal or sustained atrial fibrillation is the dominant arrhythmia and may be the sole

TABLE I.2

DISTINCTIVE FEATURES OF
GRAVES' DISEASE (TOXIC DIFFUSE GOITER)
AND PLUMMER'S DISEASE (TOXIC ADENOMATOUS GOITER)*

	GRAVES'	PLUMMER'S
Age	40 years	40 years
Onset	Acute	Insidious, slow
Goiter	Diffuse	Nodular
Bruit	Usually present	Absent
Signs & Symptoms	Usually clear-cut	Often vague, masked, sometimes apathetic
Thyroid crisis	Can occur	Rare or never
Myopathy	Yes	No
Heart Disease	Sinus tachycardia, occasional atrial fibrillation	Frequent arrhythmias, congestive failure
Ophthalmopathy	Common	Only lid retraction and lid lag
Onycholysis, pretibial	Occur, though rare	No
Lab tests	Usually diagnostic	Borderline, often equivocal
Response to iodide	Prompt	Poor, if at all
Response to antithyroid drugs	54% permanent remission	35% permanent remission
Surgery	Recurrence 2-15%	Recurrence rare
Post-therapy hypothyroidism	Common	Rare

*Modified from Schneeberg, N.G.: Essentials of Clinical Endocrinology, C.V. Mosby Co., St. Louis, Mo., p. 143, 1970.

8/ Diagnosis of Hyperthyroidism

clinical sign. Thus a therapy-resistant arrhythmia or congestive failure may be the first diagnostic hint to the diagnosis. Resistance to the action of digitalis is in part due to its shortened half-life. The ubiquity of atrial fibrillation in thyrotoxicosis in the middle-aged and elderly is well known; 10% of all obscure cases of atrial fibrillation have been found associated with hyperthyroidism. Tachycardia is almost universal in hyperthyroidism; a cardiac rate less than 80 is rare though the heart rate may exhibit great lability. The sleeping pulse rate may be of diagnostic value and is usually over 80 per minute in more than 50% of thyrotoxic patients; in euthyroid sleeping subjects a pulse rate of less than 80 is the rule.

UNUSUAL VARIETIES OF HYPERTHYROIDISM

EUTHYROID GRAVES' DISEASE

Patients who exhibit the typical ophthalmopathy of Graves' Disease but lack the clinical signs of hyperthyroidism have been called euthyroid Graves' Disease or "ophthalmopathic Graves' Disease." Thyroid function as measured by laboratory tests is generally normal but occasionally slight elevations of serum T3 have been found. RAIU is usually normal but in somewhat more than half it is non-suppressible and there is no TSH response to TRH stimulation. Antithyroid antibodies and thyroid stimulating immunoglobulins are also demonstrable in half of the cases. Findings in cases of the author are shown in Table I.3.

THYROTOXICOSIS FACTITIA

Self medication with excessive doses of a thyroid preparation should be suspected in a hyperthyroid patient without goiter or ophthalmopathy, though stare and slight lid retraction can be observed. Typical laboratory findings include low RAIU and elevated serum T4, resin T3 uptake, and FTI. If the patient is ingesting triiodothyronine (T3) serum T3 will be elevated and T4 will be suppressed. This patient is emotionally disturbed and likely to be a nurse, pharmacist, or a physician with ready access to medications. Rare examples have been reported of Graves' Disease appearing in patients who had previously received thyroid hormone therapy for hypothyroidism, infertility, irregular menses, obesity, or goiter.[5] Hyperthyroidism slowly abates when the thyroid medication is omitted. Thyrotoxicosis from thyroid medication prescribed by a physician is known as "thyrotoxicosis medicamentosa."

Diagnosis of Hyperthyroidism /9

TABLE I.3

EUTHYROID GRAVES'

Age	Sex	Duration Years	Ophthalmopathy OD mm OS (<20mm)		Goiter	RAIU 2 hr 24 hr (<6%) (10-35%)		Thyroid Scan	T3 Suppression	T4 (5-14) mg%	RT3U (25-35%)	T3 RIA (80-180) ng%	TSH RIA
59	F	8	23	17	0	15	16	N	No	N	N	--	--
35	F	7½	15	15	+	--	25	sl-enl	--	N	--	--	15.0
26	F	1	17	14	+	20 11	39 25	N	No	N	N	N	--
43	F	7½	17	15	0	22	28	N	Yes	N	N	N	2.0
46	F	6	16	19½	0	--	45	sl-enl	Yes	N	--	275	6.2
70	M	9/12	22	23	0	16	39	N	--	N	N	220	--
50	F*	6/12	21	20	0	--	32	N	--	14.0	N	N	--
41	F*	?	18	18		9.7	18.7	N	No	15.0	20%	--	--
50	F	1	22½	19½	0	--	31	--	Partial	N	N	--	--

* sisters

T3 THYROTOXICOSIS

This variety of hyperthyroidism is unique in exhibiting an elevated serum T3 with normal values for T4, RT3U, FTI, and TBG. It is not rare; Hollander[8] encountered T3 thyrotoxicosis in 4% of hyperthyroid patients in New York City; the frequency was 12.5% in Chile, an area of iodide deficiency. Normally an increased T3/T4 ratio is found in such areas thus undoubtedly making T3 thyrotoxicosis more likely to occur.

Several patients have been described with so-called "T4 thyrotoxicosis".[9] Plasma T4 is elevated but plasma T3 is normal or low. In the majority there was a serious illness in addition to hyperthyroidism which impaired the peripheral conversion of T4 to T3, a situation similar to the "low-T3-syndrome", a problem seen in ill euthyroid patients (See p. 14).

THYROIDITIS

SUBACUTE THYROIDITIS (SAT)

During the active phase follicular disruption releases T4 and T3 into the circulation and results in transient thyrotoxicosis in up to 50% of cases.[6] A variety of painless thyroiditis resembles SAT in all other characteristics but lacks a palpable, tender goiter and presents self-limited thyrotoxicosis with a low RAIU.[7]

HASHIMOTO'S THYROIDITIS (HT)

The combination of classical Graves' Disease and HT called "Hashitoxicosis", is not unexpected since they share common autoimmune characteristics. Some authors ascribe the syndrome of painless thyroiditis with transient thyrotoxicosis to HT rather than to SAT.

THYROID CARCINOMA

Hyperthyroidism rarely may derive from well differentiated follicular carcinoma of the thyroid or even from metastases, particularly after total thyroidectomy.

STRUMA OVARII

One extremely rare entity that must be considered in any hyperthyroid female without a palpable goiter and with reduced thyroid RAIU is an ovarian teratoma containing hyperfunctioning thyroid tissue.

HYPERTHYROIDISM WITH ELEVATED SERUM TSH

In hyperthyroidism the pituitary secretion of TSH is suppressed by the high circulating concentration of TH. However, a few examples of hyperthyroidism from TSH-producing pituitary tumors have been reported.[10] When there is concomitant growth hormone hypersecretion, acromegaly has been found. Elevated TSH with augmented response to TRH has been reported in a few patients either with hyperthyroidism or euthyroid Graves' Disease. The absence of a pituitary tumor makes the explanation unclear.

JODBASEDOW

Thyrotoxicosis precipitated by the administration of iodide was first observed in areas of endemic goiter where iodides were commonly employed in treatment or in prophylaxis. More recently a number of United States cases have been reported in the USA.[11] Hyperthyroidism was precipitated in four of eight patients with multinodular, non-toxic goiter who had volunteered for physiologic studies of the effects of pharmacologic doses of iodine. Hyperthyroidism has appeared in asthmatic patients receiving iodides and after diagnostic x-ray procedures utilizing iodide - containing contrast media as in urography and cholecystography.

HYPERTHYROIDISM OF TROPHOBLASTIC ORIGIN

A variety of hyperthyroidism has been encountered in women with trophoblastic tumors, either hydatidiform mole or choriocarcinoma and in men with embryonal carcinoma of the testes. In the majority clinical evidence of hyperthyroidism has been minimal or absent though several cases of severe hyperthyroidism have been described. Frequently the thyroid is not enlarged. Laboratory indices of thyroid function have been in the hyperthyroid range. In several studies increased thyroid function was noted in a large percentage of women with hydatidiform mole. Most of the evidence shows that the responsible agent is human chorionic gonadotropin (HCG), a weak thyroid stimulator.

LABORATORY FINDINGS

The laboratory diagnosis of hyperthyroidism depends on the demonstration of increased circulating T4 and T3. In addition it may be occasionally necessary to document the presence of autonomous thyroid hyperfunction to confirm the diagnosis using the thyroid suppression test. There is no perfect or all-encompassing test that can substitute for the careful opinion of a knowledgeable physician. Multiple testing is usually superfluous. In the majority of cases a single blood specimen obtained for measurement of T4, resin T3 uptake (RT3U) plus the mathematical product, the free thyroxine index (FTI), suffices to establish the diagnosis. Treatment, especially ablative surgery or irradiation with 131-I, should never be undertaken until the diagnosis is absolutely certain. In case of doubt, a therapeutic trial with an antithyroid drug or propanolol may be useful.

SERUM T4

Radioimmunoassay (RIA) has supplanted most other methods of measuring T4. Normal values range from a low of 4.5 or 5.0 mcg% to an upper limit of about 12 or 13. Values above 13 mcg% are found in more than 90% of patients with hyperthyroidism. Notable exceptions are patients with T3 thyrotoxicosis or a deficiency of TBG.

RESIN T3 UPTAKE (RT3U) AND FREE THYROXINE INDEX (FTI)

These should be determined to recognize any gross discrepancy in T4 due to abnormalities of the principal protein carrier of T4, thyroxine binding globulin (TBG). Thus in instances where TBG binding is abnormally elevated the serum T4 will be high and a false diagnosis of hyperthyroidism can be made. RT3U will be reciprocally lowered and the mathematical product, the FTI, will be normal. The most common causes for increased TBG are estrogen therapy, pregnancy (where estrogen levels are very high) and estrogen-containing contraceptive medications. Less frequent causes are infectious hepatitis, porphyria or congenital elevation of TBG. TBG-binding capacity may be depressed with androgen therapy, in the nephrotic syndrome or hepatic cirrhosis, and in congenital deficiency of TBG. In such instances the T4 will be lower than expected and the diagnosis of hyperthyroidism will be missed unless the FTI has been calculated.

It is essential in the interpretation of serum T4 values to recognize that it is the sum of bound and free T4. Most circulating T4 (99.96%) is bound to TBG and exerts no physiologic action. About 0.04% of circulating T4 is free (not bound to TBG) and is diffusable into extracellular fluids and is therefore a biologically active fraction, free to exert its effects at the cellular level. The determination of free T4 has been beyond the scope of most clinical laboratories, but recently it has become available commercially. The FTI is easily calculated, is directly proportional to FT4 and can be used therefore as an index of FT4. FTI, the mathematical product of T4 and RT3U, is most representative of the quantity of active circulating thyroid hormone and is almost invariably elevated in hyperthyroidism. Normal values for RT3U may be reported as a percentage with normals being 25-35%, or 35-45%, depending on the particular lab. A preferable method is to compare the patient's RT3U to a standard such as pooled serum from the daily lab pool. Thus RT3U patient/RT3U pooled serum equals 1 with a range of 0.8 to 1.2. Values above 1.2 are found in hyperthyroidism. A "Thyrobinding index" is the reciprocal of the above, the hyperthyroid values being at the lower end of the scale. Some laboratories report a single value for FTI, derived from the sequential determination of T4 and RT3U. The method has not gained popularity because it fails to provide serum T4 and RT3U, values that are important in making a diagnostic decision.

Thus despite divergent changes in T4 and RT3U, the FTI remains normal in euthyroid patients and is elevated only in hyperthyroidism and abnormally depressed in hypothyroidism.

Examples of T4, RT3U and FTI in hypothetical cases are shown below:

		SERUM T4 mcg/dl. (4-12)	RT3U PATIENT RT3U pooled serum (0.8-1.2)	FTI (3.2-14.4)
	Normal (euthyroid)	8	1	8.0
	Hyper-thyroidism	16	1.4	22.4
Elev. TBG	Euthyroid receiving estrogens / Pregnancy / Contraceptive pill	16	0.5	8.0
	Hypothyroidism	2.5	0.6	1.5
Low TBG	Familial Acidosis Androgens	2.5	3.2	8.0

14/ Diagnosis of Hyperthyroidism

SERUM TRIIODOTHYRONINE (T3)

The second biologically active thyroid hormone is triiodothyronine (T3). Thyroid secretion accounts for about 20% of the circulating T3; the major portion, 80%, derives from peripheral deiodination of T4. However, in hyperthyroidism the thyroidal contribution increases to 30-40% so that the normal thyroidal T4:T3 ratio of about 10:1 decreases to about 5:1. T3 is metabolically about 5 times as potent as T4, and less bound to serum proteins. Its action is more rapid but far more transient. Normal serum T3 ranges from 80-180 ng% and is almost invariably above 200 in hyperthyroidism. Though T3 is bound to TBG, abnormal binding affects it less. The preferential thyroidal secretion of T3 and the resulting three-to four-fold increase of serum T3 provides one of the most reliable tests for hyperthyroidism. Serum T3 mirrors improvement in treated thyrotoxicosis more rapidly than does serum T4 and is usually the first value to be elevated with recurrences of hyperthyroidism.

Determination of serum T3 finds its most interesting application in the diagnosis of T3 thyrotoxicosis (See p. 10). It is now well known that acutely or chronically ill patients exhibit low serum T3 values owing to an alteration in the enzyme responsible for the deiodination of T4. In this "low T3 syndrome" there is a proportional increase of reverse T3 (RT3), (3, 3', 5'-T3) a biologically inert compound. RT3 is elevated in hyperthyroidism and depressed in hypothyroidism.

Several commercial laboratories are now offering determinations of free T4 and free T3. These assays may be of additional value in patients showing alterations in TBG and in whom the diagnosis of hyperthyroidism has been equivocal.

THYROIDAL RADIOIODINE UPTAKE (RAIU)

Once a very popular laboratory modality in the diagnosis of hyperthyroidism, RAIU is used much less frequently. In toxic nodular goiter thyroid scans are essential for the recognition of the autonomous ("hot") nodule or nodules. RAIU finds its principal application today in the equivocal case where thyroid suppression tests may be of diagnostic help. It may be occasionally required to detect ectopic thyroid tissue as a rare cause of hyperthyroidism, and is of course essential in the diagnosis of the painless thyroiditis (with low RAIU). In euthyroid individuals the daily administration of 75-100 mcg of liothyronine (T3) for seven to ten days suppresses TSH and thus profoundly inhibits the ability of the thyroid gland to trap radioiodine. In hyperthyroidism TSH is already suppressed by the elevated circulating levels of T4 and T3 so that the RAIU is not altered by this dose of T3. Following a routing 24-hour RAIU the patient is given 75 mcg of T3 for seven to ten days and the RAIU is repeated. In euthyroid individuals the second uptake is reduced to less than 50% of the baseline whereas in hyperthyroidism there is no change. The test is quite reliable though failure to suppress may occur in some euthyroid subjects with nodular goiter or with autonomously functioning non-toxic adenomata. A failure to suppress may persist for long periods after apparent clinical cure of hyperthyroidism. It is sometimes used as a prognostic index of recurrence of treated thyrotoxicosis. Administration of T3 to sick or elderly patients particularly those with heart disease may provoke undesirable side effects. In patients sensitive to T3, a single 3 mg dose of sodium-L-thyroxine orally with RAIU before and seven days later has been used as a suppression test.[12]

Occasionally a low RAIU is found in a case of hyperthyroidism. Exogenous iodides will flood the extra-thyroidal pool of iodide and block thyroidal accumulation of RAI. In a variety of painless subacute thyroiditis, transient thyrotoxicosis occurs; the low RAIU found in this condition is the result of the inflammatory process together with the increased levels of circulating T4 and T3 suppressing TSH. With low RAIU and hyperthyroidism one must also consider unusual thyroid sites as struma ovarii, lingual thyroid, or the more caudad locations of a substernal goiter.

THYROTROPHIN RELEASING HORMONE TEST (TRH)

In normal subjects the intravenous administration of 200-500 mcg of TRH promotes a rise of serum TSH from $5-25\ \mu U/ml$ within 20 to 30 minutes. In hyperthyroidism this response does not occur; a significant TRH induced rise of TSH would constitute strong evidence against the diagnosis of hyperthyroidism. The test is safer and less time consuming than the T3 suppression test and may completely supplant it. Its principle drawback is the need for an intravenous infusion which may require hospitalization where out-patient facilities are lacking. TRH can be employed by intramuscular injection or even orally but much larger doses of this expensive hormone are necessary.

SUMMARY OF THE LABORATORY DIAGNOSIS OF HYPERTHYROIDISM

1. Determine serum T4, RT3U and FTI.

2. If #1 is normal or equivocal do serum T3 (RIA) to detect borderline hyperthyroidism or T3-thyrotoxicosis.

3. If #1 and #2 are indeterminate do RAIU and T3 suppression test (or single dose T4 suppression test), or TRH stimulation test. In nodular goiter do a thyroid scan.

4. Other biochemical and physiological changes occur from the impact of thyroid hormones on peripheral tissue but are of limited diagnostic value. These are:

    a) serum cholesterol - decreased
    b) Achilles reflex time - shortened
    c) BMR-increased
    d) Serum calcium-elevated (15% of patients)
    e) CPK-often reduced
    f) Sex-steroid-binding-protein-increased
    g) Erythrocyte glucose-6-phosphate dehydrogenase, carbonic anhydrase, sodium and zinc increased
    h) Serum thyroglobulin often increased
    i) Timing of Korotkoff arterial sounds with the QRS complex of the ECG. [13]

REFERENCES

1. Crooks, EJ, Murray, IPC, Wayne, EJ: Statistical methods applied to the clinical diagnosis of thyrotoxicosis. Quart J Med 28:211, 1959.

2. Werner, SC, Coleman, J and Franzen, LA: Ultrasonographic evidence of a consistent orbital involvement in Graves' Disease. New Eng J Med 190:144, 1974.

3. Werner, SC: Classification of the eye changes of Graves' Disease. J Clin Endocrinol & Metab 29:982, 1969.

4. Werner, SC: Eye changes. In: The Thyroid, A Fundamental and Clinical Text, 4th edition. S.C. Werner and S.H. Ingbar (Eds.), Harper and Row, New York, 1978, pp. 655-659.

5. Dymling, JP, and Becker, DV: Occurrence of hyperthyroidism in patients receiving thyroid hormone. J Clin Endocrinol & Metab 27:1487, 1967.

6. Volpe, R: Acute and subacute thyroiditis. Pharmac Ther C 1;171, 1976.

7. Dorfman, SG, Cooperman, MT, Nelson, RL, et al.: Painless thyroiditis and transient hyperthyroidism without goiter. Ann Intern Med 86:24, 1977.

8. Hollander, CS, Mitsuma, T, Shenkman, L, et al.: T3-Toxicosis in an iodine-deficient area. Lancet 2:1276, 1972.

9. Joasoa, A: T4 Thyrotoxicosis with normal or low serum T3 concentration. Aust N Z J Med 5:432, 1975.

10. Huff, TA: Disorders Leading to TSH hypersecretion. In: The Pituitary A Current Review, MB Allen, Jr. and V.B. Mahech, Academic Press, New York, 1977, p. 169.

11. Vagenakis, AG, Wang, GA, Burger, A, et al.: Iodine-induced thyrotoxicosis in Boston. New Eng J Med 287:523, 1972.

12. Wenzel, KW, and Meinhold, H: Evidence of lower toxicity during thyroxine suppression after a single 3 mg 1-thyroxine dose: Comparison to the classical 1-triiodothyronine test for thyroid suppressibility. J Clin Endocrinol & Metab 38: 902, 1974.

13. Rodbard, D, Fujita, T, & Rodbard, S: Esimation of thyroid function by timing the arterial sounds. JAMA, 201: 884, 1977.

CHAPTER II

TREATMENT OF HYPERTHYROIDISM: GENERAL CONSIDERATIONS

In discussing the treatment of hyperthyroidism it is helpful to consider the available modalities as either definitive or symptomatic. The definitive modalities--radioiodine ablation, subtotal thyroidectomy, or a thioamide--will control the symptoms of hyperthyroidism and may produce a permanent remission of the disease. Symptomatic agents--reserpine, guanethidine, propranolol, or iodine--will control the manifestations of the disease but will not produce a permanent remission. Ablation with radioiodine or subtotal thyroidectomy destroys a portion of the thyroid; a thioamide temporarily blocks the synthesis of the thyroid hormones. None of these definitive modalities can said to have been selected because of considerations which fit more recent concepts about the etiology of hyperthyroidism. Remission occurs because sufficient thyroid has been destroyed by radioiodine or surgery or because the remission persists after the course of a thioamide has been completed. Any speculation about pathophysiological mechanism rarely enters into the choice of a definitive therapy for Graves' Disease. The overactive nodular thyroid does require some special thought in the selection of therapy. On the other hand adrenergic blocking agents were introduced because the sympathetic nervous system was thought to be involved in the production of the symptoms of hyperthyroidism. There is little evidence to support this contention yet such agents are quite useful in controlling the symptoms of hyperthyroidism.

Each of the definitive modalities differ in the sequence with which immediate and permanent control is achieved and the time required to reach these goals. One of the thioamides will control the symptoms within a period of six weeks, yet therapy is continued for at least one year before stopping the medication to decide if the remission will be permanent. Thioamides control the symptoms rapidly but are the slowest in terms of the time elapsed between diagnosis and permanent remission. Before proceeding with subtotal thyroidectomy it is necessary to control the hyperthyroidism with either a thioamide or propranolol. Immediate control of the thyrotoxicosis requires three to six weeks with one of these agents before permanent control is attempted with subtotal thyroidectomy, another modality; yet the time from diagnosis to permanent remission will often be as short as three months. Though radioiodine can be administered as soon as the diagnosis of hyperthyroidism is established, permanent control may not be evident for a minimum of two to three months. In this interval temporary control of the symptoms is sometimes necessary using either a thioamide or propranolol. The time between diagnosis and permanent remission will be no shorter than three months and will often be as long as six months to one year. Subsequent chapters will discuss these various modalities in detail.

These three modalities vary in the rate of permanent remission and the incidence of hypothyroidism. Nearly all patients respond to radioiodine although several doses may be necessary. Subtotal thyroidectomy produces a permanent remission in perhaps 90% of patients, a course of thioamides in only 30-40%. Hypothyroidism when produced by a thioamide will disappear when the drug is stopped. The incidence of permanent hypothyroidism after radioiodine is at least 15% after the first year of followup and increases by 3-4% thereafter. After surgery about 30-40% of patients become hypothyroid.

Thioamides are easy to administer and to adjust. Any one of these compounds control the symptoms in a matter of weeks. Side effects are rare and usually disappear quickly. Successful therapy does demand careful patient compliance for the entire course of therapy. Surgery requires the briefest period of patient compliance but introduces the complications of surgery. These include such problems as damage to the parathyroids, damage to the recurrent and superior laryngeal nerves, postoperative bleeding and laryngeal edema. Administration of radioiodine is no more difficult than the ingestion of a capsule containing the isotope. This simplicity must be balanced by such considerations as the induction of thyroid carcinoma, leukemia, and gonadal damage and the high incidence of subsequent hypothyroidism.

Symptomatic control may be necessary under many circumstances. Often symptoms are so severe that control is necessary before the definitive modality becomes effective. Thus until radioiodine ablation succeeds, propranolol or a thioamide can provide temporary, symptomatic relief. Or the patient may be sufficiently ill so that even the six weeks for the improvement with thioamides may be too long and propranolol will be necessary to control symptoms. It must be stressed, too, that before surgery can be undertaken, control of the hyperthyroidism must be attained with a thioamide or propranolol. The selection of the agent for symptomatic control in these circumstances will be discussed in detail in Chapter III, Part II. Suffice it to note that propranolol has become the most widely used agent for reduction of symptoms. Its effect appears within a matter of minutes with the intravenous route, and within a matter of hours given orally. Its reliability and safety are far superior to the other adrenergic agents--reserpine and guanethidine. Iodine is used to control symptoms only in thyroid storm. Although the thioamides are not selected as often recently as definitive agents, any one is still useful in the control of symptoms.

The selection of a therapy for hyperthyroidism can also be considered in terms of any of the following categories: (1) specific manifestations of the disease, (2) characteristics of the thyroid enlargement, (3) the presence of concurrent medical problems, or (4) age of the patient. Chapter VII discusses the treatment of thyroid storm, hyperthyroidism in pregnancy, apathetic hyperthyroidism, thyroid ophthalmopathy, and several unusual forms of hyperthyroidism. The treatment of hyperthyroidism in children is reviewed in Chapter VI.

The age of the patient is always a consideration in deciding the minimum age at which the use of radioiodine is appropriate. Although there has been favorable experience with radioiodine in children most physicians prefer to use it only in patients over thirty and some will not administer it in patients under forty. As will be noted in subsequent discussions there is little support for the fear of the production of thyroid carcinoma, or leukemia. Nor is there any substantial evidence that congenital anomalies appear more frequently in the offspring of patients so treated. Gonadal irradiation for that matter is probably no greater than such radiological procedures as an intravenous pyelogram or a barium enema. The selection of a minimum age more often than not stems from a desire to restrict radioiodine to the relatively older patient. In this way the lag in the appearance of such complications will lessen the risk or at least minimize it. In a sense time is on the side of the patient. Whatever the evidence might be it is often difficult to dispell the fears of radiation for patients in the reproductive years. It is the preference of the author to use radioiodine as the first choice in patients over forty and to use it whenever possible in patients over thirty. For most patients in the age range of twenty to thirty, and for a substantial proportion of patients thirty to forty subtotal thyroidectomy will be the most appropriate modality for definitive therapy. A thioamide is usually not an attractive alternative since it requires close patient cooperation and the incidence of permanent remissions is so disappointing. The most recent data as reviewed in Chapter III, Part I indicates that less than 40% of patients remain in remission after a course of a thioamide for one year and after subsequent years it is far less. For most patients a thioamide only delays the choice of surgery or radioiodine.

The characteristics of the thyroid as the distinction between Graves' Disease and Plummer's Disease are often used to determine the most appropriate modality of therapy. Many physicians favor subtotal thyroidectomy for the treatment of the toxic nodular goiter. Chapter V and VI discuss the merits of these arguments in terms of the overall use of radioiodine and surgery. There is ample evidence that radioiodine is quite effective in nodular goiters and is in many cases far safer. Proponents of surgery argue that these nodular thyroids are far more resistant to any therapy and are usually quite resistant to radioiodine. Another argument is that since patients with nodular goiters are often seriously ill the rapidity of the production of euthyroidism with surgery represents a distinct advantage over the other modalities. Yet by controlling the manifestations of hyperthyroidism with a thioamide the situation is less desperate and there is then ample time for ablation with radioiodine. Maintaining euthyroidism with the thioamide prevents a recurrence of the hyperthyroidism until the radioiodine proves effective. Either approach has yielded favorable results in skilled hands. It is the author's preference to select radioiodine according to age. Large thyroids, most unusual in hyperthyroidism, will not reliably diminish in size with either radioiodine or a thioamide so then when size is a consideration then surgery is indicated. And whenever the features of the thyroid raise the suspicion of a co-existing carcinoma, surgery is necessary to resolve the problem.

22/ Treatment of Hyperthyroidism

The clinical presentation of thyrotoxicosis can vary considerably. Thyroid storm is a medical emergency that requires aggressive therapy if the patient is to survive. The details of therapy are discussed in Chapter VII. For most other patients a decision about definitive therapy will be influenced only in part by the exact combination of symptoms. A case in point is apathetic hyperthyroidism, a form of hyperthyroidism in which the patient is anything but hyperkinetic. Although it may appear that the illness is far more benign than the usual form of hyperthyroidism such is not the case. Therapy must be planned in the same manner as it would be in the usual hyperkinetic patient with the full complement of symptoms. Much the same is true of occult hyperthyroidism in which the disease is manifested as abnormalities within a single organ system. Thus atrial fibrillation may be the sole sign of the disease yet therapy must be chosen with the same care as if other signs and symptoms were present. For the older patient with a concurrent illness as congestive heart failure it may be necessary to control the hyperthyroidism with a thioamide before administering a therapeutic dose of radioiodine. This permits depletion of the stores of thyroid hormones and should avoid the risks of sudden release of hormones with a radiation thyroiditis. Chapter V discusses the problems of exacerbation of hyperthyroidism with the use of radioiodine.

Several concurrent problems may influence the choice of therapy. Hyperthyroidism in pregnancy presents many dilemmas which are considered in Chapter VIII. In younger patients the presence of a serious cardiac problem as a valvular lesion or a disease as Sickle Cell Disease will often make radioiodine the best choice of definitive therapy. Thyroid ophthalmopathy has been used to select one definitive modality over another or to dictate the rapidity with which the hyperthyroidism is controlled. Chapter VII will review the subject in more detail. In most circumstances it is far preferable to control the hyperthyroidism as rapidly as possible since most surgical procedures on the eye require that the hyperthyroidism be controlled first. With skillful use of the available agents neither hyperthyroidism or its control should interfere with the treatment of concurrent medical problems.

CHAPTER III

DRUG THERAPY OF HYPERTHYROIDISM

There are several applications for drugs in the treatment of hyperthyroidism. Thioamides such as propylthiouracil (PTU) or methimazole (MMI) can be used to control the symptoms of hyperthyroidism and when given over a prolonged period are often followed by a permanent remission of the disease. Agents such as propranolol, reserpine, guanethidine, and phenobarbital are often added to one of the definitive modalities of therapy to produce rapid relief of the symptoms of hyperthyroidism. Iodides are employed in the treatment of thyroid storm and to produce involution of the overactive thyroid prior to subtotal thyroidectomy. Even though all of these drugs have been used for the control of the symptoms of hyperthyroidism the mechanism of action varies. The effects of PTU and MMI are achieved by blocking the synthesis of the thyroid hormones. The adrenergic-blocking agents as propranolol, reserpine and guanethidine interfere with the peripheral effects of the thyroid hormones. Iodides block the release of thyroid hormones from the thyroid. In addition it may produce the hypervascularity of the thyroid by increasing the volume of colloid. Thioamides are discussed in Part One of this chapter; the other agents are discussed in Part Two.

24/ Drug Therapy of Hyperthyroidism

PART ONE: THIOAMIDES

A discussion of the drugs used to produce a permanent remission of hyperthyroidism is in essence a review of the group of thioamide compounds. More potent members of the group are actually thioureylenes. Figure 3.1 shows the common thioamide and thioureylene structure as well as several derivatives. Through experience those thioamides as thiouracil which have unquestioned toxicity have been dropped so that the choice of a specific agent now rests more on custom than for any other specific reason. All of the thioamides are remarkably similar with regard to effectiveness in controlling the hyperthyroidism, the incidence of side effects, and the mechanism of action. The present discussion will be limited to PTU and MMI, the two thioamides in use in the United States. For comparison carbimazole, a thioamide used in several other countries, is also depicted in Figure 3.1. Perchlorate is sometimes mentioned in discussion of therapy as an alternative to a thioamide, but the occurrence of fatal asplastic anemia precludes its use except for diagnostic purposes.[1]

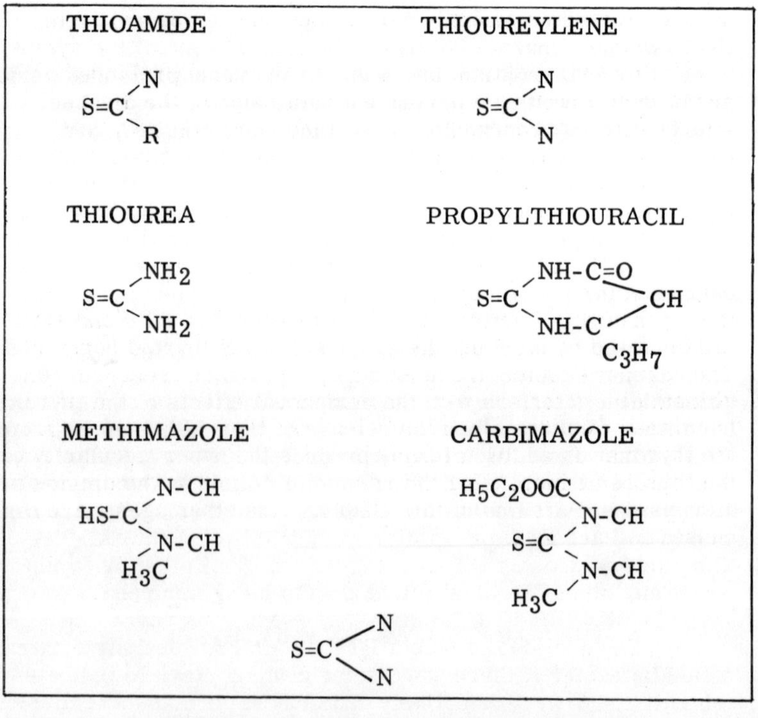

FIGURE 3.1: Structure of thioamides

DEFINITIVE THERAPY

The limited possibilities for a permanent remission following a course of a year or more of a thioamide make PTU or MMI a rather unsatisfactory choice as a definitive agent. Discussions favoring this approach would usually cite a value of 55% as the expected incidence of permanent remission,[2] although values were reported from as high as 82% to as low as 41%.[3,4] Since the duration of therapy in these reports varied from one to several years and the follow-up ranged from one year to more than ten, comparison of such experience was quite difficult. Furthermore when the rates of permanent remission from individual reports in the decade from 1962 to 1972 were arranged by the year of the reports, it became clear that there was a continual fall in the incidence of permanent remission.[5] The incidence of permanent remission after one year of therapy in this 1973 report was a dissappointing 13.6%. It is probably fair at present to place the estimate of permanent remission following the use of a thioamide for one year at 24%.[5a] Continuation of the medication for an additional one year will probably produce a permanent remission in about 20% of the remaining patients.

An explanation for this fall in remission remains unclear. It has been suggested that the patients in several reports were weighted towards those patients who would have been most likely to respond to a thioamide.[5a] On the other hand many lines of evidence point toward a rise in dietary iodine as the reason for this change.[5] It had been demonstrated, for example, that if patients were placed on an iodine supplement following a course of thioamide therapy recurrences occurred more often and sooner than in a control group without the supplement.[6] The strength of this line of reasoning was weakened by the observation that the remission in an area of low iodine intake was still only 32%.[7] One might argue that a permanent remission with a thioamide reflects only the spontaneous remission of hyperthyroidism. Observations from the early part of this century indicated that about 30% of hyperthyroid patients underwent a spontaneous remission.[8] Allowing for limitations in the diagnosis of hyperthyroidism 50 to 60 years ago, this rate of spontaneous remission seems quite similar to that following thioamides. Certainly at present there is no evidence that these thioamides exert any other thyroidal effect than to block hormonal synthesis.

The decision to select PTU or MMI for definitive therapy would be easier if there were some clinical clues to indicate which patients were most likely to undergo a permanent remission.

Considered helpful are small thyroid size, diffuse thyroid enlargement, symptoms present for less than a year, the occurrence of T3 thyrotoxicosis, or the absence of HLA antigens. [9, 10, 11] The usefulness of these clues requires some qualification. Most patients experience the symptoms of hyperthyroidism for less than a year before the diagnosis is made. Patients with a longer history have usually learned to tolerate their symptoms quite well and will often fail to take medication with any degree of regularity. Thus control of the hyperthyroidism is not achieved. In addition several years of undetected hyperthyroidism may make the initial diagnosis difficult and the response to therapy even harder to evaluate, needlessly delaying the cure. As to characteristics of the thyroid, evaluation of the size of the thyroid and its configuration rests largely on the examiner's skill and background. Conclusions along these lines are subjective at best. Remission does occur more frequently when the thyroid decreases significantly in size even with the vagueness of such terminology. However, drug therapy cannot be planned on this basis alone since the observation is possible only after therapy has been started. Very large thyroids are unusual in untreated hyperthyroidism and do not decrease rapidly enough or sufficiently enough with thioamides to recommend this form of therapy. Although T3 thyrotoxicosis differs in its laboratory presentation, its clinical manifestations are not sufficiently different from the conventional forms of hyperthyroidism to justify that it will respond differently to therapy. Somewhat more promising is the correlation of the response to thioamides and the absence of HLA-B8.[11] It was suggested that the presence of HLA-B8 indicated the persistence of a thyrotropin-receptor stimulating antibody and hence the failure of therapy. This may then provide a means of identifying the patient who will remain in remission following a course of thioamide.

It has been customary to administer PTU or MMI at intervals of six or eight hours for the duration of therapy, although experimental data to support this was quite slim. Recent measurements of plasma levels of PTU or MMI have demonstrated comparable periods for the effect of a thioamide and lend support to the need for regularly spaced medication.[12, 13, 14] Whether or not the block of the thyroid hormone synthesis persists as levels of thioamide falls remains unsolved. Fluctuating plasma levels might not reflect corresponding changes in the degree of block of thyroid hormone synthesis. It seemed promising to attempt to achieve control of the hyperthyroidism and to induce a permanent remission with a single, daily dose of PTU or MMI.[9, 15] The initial success with this mode of administration was not confirmed and it became clear that repeated doses at six or eight hourly intervals were necessary.[16] The advantage of better patient cooperation with a single dose sacrificed effective control of the hyperthyroidism. As the course of treatment proceeds it is often possible to reduce the dose of PTU or MMI or increase the interval between doses and still maintain control. This contrasts with beginning therapy which requires administration of the medication at more frequent intervals. As treatment continues plasma levels of PTU persist longer and longer, [12] perhaps extending the thyroid effect even longer and reducing the need for frequent doses.

Just as customary as regularly spaced doses of thioamide is the practice of continuing therapy for a minimum of one year. The need for this interval has been questioned.[17] By continuing MMI only until euthyroidism was first achieved, the incidence of permanent remission after a two-year follow up compared favorably with the use of MMI for a full year. The duration of therapy averaged four to five months. This approach might well help to solve the dilemma of the low rate of permanent remission. Rather than commit a patient to a full year of MMI or PTU, a four or five month course would be used. Patients who failed to respond by undergoing a permanent remission could then be directed more quickly to either surgery or radioiodine. A note of caution recently indicated some doubt about the success of this approach.[42]

To decide if the remission of the disease is permanent the presence of normal thyroid suppression has been employed instead of simply waiting for the recurrence of the symptoms. Various techniques of suppression have been tried either during the course of therapy with a thioamide[15] or once the course has been completed.[18] Determination of suppressibility of the thyroid involves measurement of thyroid iodine uptake while the patient takes exogenous thyroid in one form or another. If thyroid function is normal it and the pituitary will respond so that the exogenous hormone will produce a depression of the uptake of iodine. Exact values will depend on the form of thyroid supplement used, the duration of administration of the exogenous thyroid, and the interval chosen for measurement of uptake. There are many limitations to the application of this test. Most techniques have used thyroid iodine uptake at one half hour following the administration of the tracer. This requires an intravenous preparation of radioactive iodine, a form not often available. In patients who have not undergone a permanent remission the addition of exogenous thyroid, by adding more hormone, sometimes produces quite severe symptoms. Techniques which use several weeks of thyroid suppression are much too cumbersome to be helpful. It is far easier to treat the patient either until euthyroidism occurs or for a full year and then consider another form of definitive therapy with the first evidence of recurrence of the hyperthyroidism.

The question also arises as to the advisability of repeating thioamide therapy if permanent remission fails to occur after one year of therapy. Irrespective of the experience the incidence of remission is highest after one year of therapy. Successive years of therapy add smaller numbers to the overall rate of remission. For example, in one series a permanent remission was achieved in 56% of the patients after a single year of therapy. In the remaining hyperthyroid patients only 36% remained in remission after an additional year of therapy and only 25% after two years.[19] This hardly raises much enthusiasm for a course of a thioamide for longer than one year. Most recurrences will appear within twelve to eighteen months after therapy. The rates of recurrence are highest in the first few months following the discontinuation of the thioamide and then begin to plateau as eighteen months approaches. Hence for most patients the best results are achieved with one year of therapy and most recurrences occur within the following year.

MECHANISM OF ACTION

Although many theories have been offered to explain the effects of the thioamides, it seems quite likely that the problem is far more complex than the interference with thyroid hormone synthesis at a single step in the pathway. The effects of thioamides depend on the concentration of the thioamide in the plasma, the concentration of the iodide within the thyroid, the severity of the hyperthyroidism, the metabolism of thioamides, and the duration of thioamide therapy. To help in understanding these several theories, an outline of thyroid hormone formation is shown in Table III.1.

One view is that the coupling step is most sensitive to PTU.[20] Thus in animal experiments as the dose of PTU is increased the concentrations of triiodothyronine (T3) and thyroxine (T4) fall in thyroid homoginates before the concentrations of monoiodotyrosine (MIT) and diiodotyrosine (DIT). Although just a postulate this would explain the observation that during the administration of a thioamide the uptake of iodine by the thyroid is not as fully depressed at 30 minutes as it is at 24 hours.[21] Since coupling is blocked the initial uptake reflects entry into MIT and DIT and the later uptakes a diminished thyroid production of T3 and T4.[22] Another intriguing postulate is that the thioamides or a subsequent metabolite bind to thyroglobulin and in this manner prevent the coupling reaction.[23]

TABLE III.1.

STEPS IN THYROID HORMONE SYNTHESIS

STEP	COMMENT
Iodine Trapping	Blocked with perchlorate
Organification	Introduction of iodine into tyrosyl residue: Formation of MIT, DIT
Coupling	Formation of T3, T4
Storage in thyroglobulin	
Release of T3, T4 from celloid into plasma	Blocked with iodide
MIT-Monoiodotyrosing DIT-Diiodotyrosine	T3-Triiodothyronine T4-Thyroxine

Other theories have involved the effect on thyroid peroxidase, an enzyme which catalyzes the transformation of iodine into a more active form and also catalyzes the introduction of this active form onto the tyrosyl residue. It has been suggested that thioamides block the activation of iodine,[24] or on the other hand act as a competitive inhibitor of peroxidase.[25] A synthesis of these viewpoints holds that the thioamides in competition with iodine inhibit the formation of the active form of iodine and are in turn oxidized by this active species.[26] From the clinical standpoint at lower plasma levels a thioamide may not fully block formation of the active form of iodine but through its oxidation by this active form it interferes with the production of the thyroid hormones. Thus increasing the dose of a thioamide may not actually increase the intrathyroid concentration of the drug but simply increase its intrathyroidal metabolism.[26a]

Until recently, provided that toxicity remained within safe limits, one thioamide was considered interchangeable with another. Whether PTU or MMI was selected the final outcome differed little. Along with the discovery that an important step in the action of the thyroid hormones consisted of the peripheral conversion of T4 and T3 was the fact that PTU but not MMI inhibited this conversion.[27, 28, 29] Thus PTU might block the formation of T3 and could provide more effective control of the symptoms of hyperthyroidism. In pregnancy since all thioamides cross the placental barrier such an effect might reduce T3 available to the fetus and diminish the effects of thyroid hormone at the cellular level.

COMPLICATIONS OF THIOAMIDES

The more common side effects occur in perhaps 5% of patients taking PTU or MMI and include a variety of skin eruptions, leukopenia, agranulocytosis, or serum sickness-like reactions. A tabulation of less common complications is contained in Table III. 2. Early estimates of the incidence of the occurrence of side effects suggested that MMI might be somewhat more toxic than PTU.[30] However, the overall use of MMI was far less than that of PTU. With regard to more catastrophic complications, an informal survey[31] among endocrinologists in the Philadelphia area placed the incidence of agranulocytosis at 1.8% with PTU and 0.6% with MMI. Aplatic anemia occurred once in several thousand cases with either drug. Judging from many reported cases in general, the expected incidence of agranulocytosis is probably closer to 0.1%.[32] Fatalities are fortunately even more unusual.

The etiology of these untoward reaction with conventional doses of MMI and PTU is undoubtedly a hypersensitivity reaction. With a dose of MMI of 120 mg/day, roughly twice the usual highest recommended dose, toxic reactions occur with alarming frequency and are probably dose related.[42] This fact must be kept in mind when large doses of MMI or for that matter PTU are contemplated. Most side effects appear within the first few weeks of therapy and disappear promptly when the offending drug is withdrawn. However, some complications do not fit this pattern. Jaundice which appears with the use of MMI often will not clear for as long as two months following withdrawal of the drug.[40]

Without a means to predict which patient is at risk for these complications prompt recognition becomes imperative. There is no substitute for an alert physician. There is usually little choice but to stop the offending medication. Only if leukopenia can be attributed to the hyperthyroidism itself is continuance of PTU or MMI warranted. Most reactions disappear without further therapy but in severe reaction more aggressive steps are required. For serum sickness corticosteroids may be necessary. For agranulocytosis the usual measures of isolation and antibiotics are ordinarily followed by recovery. The

TABLE III. 2.

ADVERSE REACTIONS WITH PTU AND MMI

System Involved	Specific Reaction	Agent	Reference
1. Hematologic	a) Granulocytopenia (and lupus-like syndrome)	PTU	33
	b) Granulocytopenia anemia hemolytic	PTU	34
	c) Aplastic anemia	MMI	31, 35
	d) Bone marrow aplasia	PTU	36
	e) Hypoprothrombinemia	PTU	38
	g) Operative bleeding	PTU	39
2. Connective Tissue	a) Arthritis	MMI	37
	b) Collogen-like syndrome	PTU MMI	41
3. Hepatic	a) Jaundice	MMI	40

32/ Drug Therapy of Hyperthyroidism

decision to switch to the other thioamide is difficult. The availability of alternatives as ^{131}I, or subtotal thyroidectomy with propranolol and iodine preparation make the use of another thioamide less attractive than in the past. Many physicians will start the other thioamide at a very low dose and then slowly increase until the full therapeutic level is reached.

The following case illustrates the problem of toxicity of the thioamides. The patient, a 17-year-old woman, had noted nervousness, irritability, palpitations, and increased sweating for about nine months before the diagnosis of hyperthyroidism was made in June, 1975. She was placed on MMI and over the first two weeks of therapy her symptoms began to decrease. Toward the end of June a maculopapular rash appeared. There was some relief from the pruritis with the addition of diphenhydramine but the MMI was not stopped. In early July recurrent arthralgias appeared and over the month became increasingly severe. At the end of July prednisone was started and the MMI stopped. She had numerous joints involved, was febrile, and had severe malaise.

In early August, 1975, the arthritis and the skin eruption disappeared so that rapid withdrawal of the prednisone was possible. Her weight was 121 pounds, and pulse 140/minute. The thyroid was twice normal in size. There was a tremor of her hands and her palms were warm and moist. The white blood cell count was 13,800, hemoglobin 13.3%, and hematocrit 39.9%. On differential there were 67% polymorphonuclear cells, 28% lymphocytes, 4% monocytes and 1% eosinophiles. A T4 was 13.4 mcgm% (normal less than 12 mcgm%). In September, 1975, PTU was introduced beginning at 25 mg daily. Her symptoms were controlled with phenobarbital and reserpine. By November the dose of PTU had reached 100 mg daily in divided doses. Her weight was then 135 pounds and her pulse 65/minute. The tremor had disappeared but the thyroid size remained unchanged. The T4 was 4.5 mcgm%. From November onward it was possible to maintain control of the hyperthyroidism with PTU alone.

The first evidence of toxicity, a drug eruption, appeared quite benign at first, and thus the MMI was not stopped. The development of serum sickness required the use of prednisone and left no choice about continuation of the MMI. Had the problem occurred within the last year or two the patient would more likely have been admitted to the hospital as soon as the drug reaction subsided, and prepared for surgery with a combination of propranolol and iodine. In a somewhat older patient ^{131}I

Drug Therapy of Hyperthyroidism /33

would have been the preferred alternative. The patient declined ^{131}I therapy so that only substitution with PTU remained. In 1975 propranolol was not yet used to prepare patients for subtotal thyroidectomy. Fortunately the course thereafter was quite satisfactory and her symptoms, which had improved on MMI, showed a similar response to PTU. The case should also point out that reactions with either PTU or MMI although not life threatening can be quite incapacitating. It seems most prudent to stop the offending drug regardless of how mild a drug reaction might be.

SPECIFICS OF THERAPY WITH THIOAMIDES

The uses of either MMI or PTU include the following:

1) As definitive therapy
2) As a means of preparing patients for surgery
3) As an adjunct to ^{131}therapy
4) As a component in the management of thyroid storm

Either PTU or MMI is still appropriate to prepare the hyperthyroid patient for subtotal thyroidectomy. It is customary to render the patient euthyroid before surgery. By using a dose of 100 mg PTU or 10 mg MMI every 8 hours it is usually possible to achieve euthyroidism within 6 weeks. With the more toxic patient it will sometimes be necessary to increase the size of the dose to 200 mg of PTU or 20 mg of MMI or even decrease the interval to 6 hours between doses. Once the patient is euthyroid by clinical findings and laboratory tests, surgery can be scheduled. To reduce the vascularity of the gland it is necessary to add an iodide solution as Lugol's Solution about one week before surgery. In contrast, preparation for surgery with propranolol requires only two to three weeks, however, the continued risk of thyroid storm still make a thioamide a preferred means of preparation. Propranolol should be reserved for those situations in which a thioamide is not practical as in the uncooperative patient or when time is of the essence.

By combining MMI or PTU with ^{131}I ablation, the control of hyperthyroidism is far more effective, especially since radioiodine requires three months on the average for the full effect to appear. Once the ablative dose of radioiodine is administered, PTU or MMI can be added and continued until it is time to decide if a second dose will be necessary. In this scheme the thioamide is started within 3-6 days after the dose of ^{131}I and continued for roughly 10 weeks. The persistence of an elevated thyroid iodine uptake will indicate whether or not another ablative dose of ^{131}I will be necessary. Symptoms of hyperthyroidism should disappear with the course of the thioamide so that the patient will not have to experience this discomfort until the radioiodine proves effective. This aspect of thioamides is considered in more detail in Chapter V.

Special consideration of the treatment of hyperthyroidism in pregnancy and childhood are covered in Chapters VII and VI respectively. The management of thyroid storm is discussed in Chapter VII.

The selection of MMI or PTU as a definitive agent must be considered in the light of the low frequency of permanent remissions as well as the need to take the medication regularly for as long as one year. In childhood and in the pregnant patient the choice is still weighed toward thioamides. For the patients between age twenty and forty, often the fear of radioiodine and the unwillingness to undergo a surgical procedure provides the reasons for choosing the drug. One clear advantage of PTU or MMI is that since the drug effect disappears with cessation of the drug, a switch to another modality is always possible.

The usual guidelines for the initial dose of MMI are 10 to 20 mg every 6 or 8 hours and for PTU 100 to 200 mg every 6 or 8 hours. A dose of 25 mg MMI every six hours will produce a full block of the synthesis of hormones;[43] unfortunately at this dose toxic reactions occur with alarming frequency.[42] There is recent evidence that a full block probably is not required to produce control of the hyperthyroidism.[26a] It is best to begin with 10 mg of MMI or 100 mg of PTU every 8 hours. The dose may be increased after one month if improvement fails to occur. It is often sufficient to administer the dose at six hours intervals. A rapidly deteriorating clinical setting often requires doubling the dose of PTU to 200 mg of MMI to 20 mg every 8 hours. As improvement occurs the frequency of the dose can be reduced to every 12 hours and if necessary the size of the dose can be reduced. Improvement will be reflected in the improvement of symptoms and signs and the return of the parameters of thyroid function to normal. It requires about 6 weeks to 3 months for the patient to become euthyroid. Unfortunately measurements of T3 have limited value since PTU a fall occurs within a matter of days after thioamide therapy has started.[44] Clinical impression should be supported by measurements of T4, however, the improvement in clinical findings may lag behind the fall in the T4.[45]

The question often arises as to why patients fail to respond to PTU or MMI. Explanations include failure to take medication, an unusually rapid inactivation of thioamides, or an inability to rapidly deplete thyroid hormone stores. In most circumstances the patient just fails to take the medication. The following case illustrates this problem.

The patient, a 21-year-old woman, was first evaluated for hyperthyroidism in April, 1978. A T4 was 23 mcg% (normal less than 12 mcgm%) and T3 resin, 33% (normal 25-35%). A 24-hour thyroid uptake with ^{131}I was 95%. Between April and September the patient failed to respond to therapy although the dose of PTU was increased to 100 mg every 6 hours. Her weight remained at 112 pounds, her pulse above 90/minute and the thyroid at two to three times normal in size. To judge the effectiveness of thioamide therapy a perchlorate washout test was performed. As shown in Table III.3 the administration of one gram of perchlorate orally 50 minutes after the dose of ^{131}I and 12 hours after 100 mg of PTU discharged some of the radioactivity already accumulated. If hormone synthesis is blocked, then iodine cannot proceed beyond the iodine trap, and perchlorate should discharge the iodine from the trap. Had PTU not been effective, radioactivity would not fall, reflecting the lack of block of thyroid hormone synthesis. The lack of response to PTU clearly resulted from a failure of the patient to taker her medication. Altering the dose schedule or changing the medication or combining therapy would prove futile. The availability of propranolol permits preparation of such patients for surgery under inpatient supervision. The perchlorate test can help in deciding about continuing thioamide therapy or choosing another modality. Avoiding unnecessary delay provides the most satisfactory treatment of the hyperthyroidism.

The successful use of MMI as definitive therapy to produce a permanent remission is illustrated by the following case. In December, 1973, the patient, a 28-year-old male, complained of nervousness, irritability, increased sweating, pruritis, insomnia, and a ten pound weight loss. There were visible muscle tremors at rest, his pulse was 104/minute and the thyroid twice normal in size. A T4 and 14 mcgm% (normal 4-12 mcgm%) and thyroid uptake at 24 hours with ^{131}I 52%. The patient was started on MMI 10 mg every eight hours and propranolol 10 mg every six hours.

In January, 1974, his symptoms had decreased somewhat, his weight had increased by three pounds but the tremors persisted. In March, 1974, his weight had increased by ten pounds and all symptoms had disappeared. The size of the thyroid remained unchanged. A T4 was 2.5 mcgm% (normal 4-12

36/ Drug Therapy of Hyperthyroidism

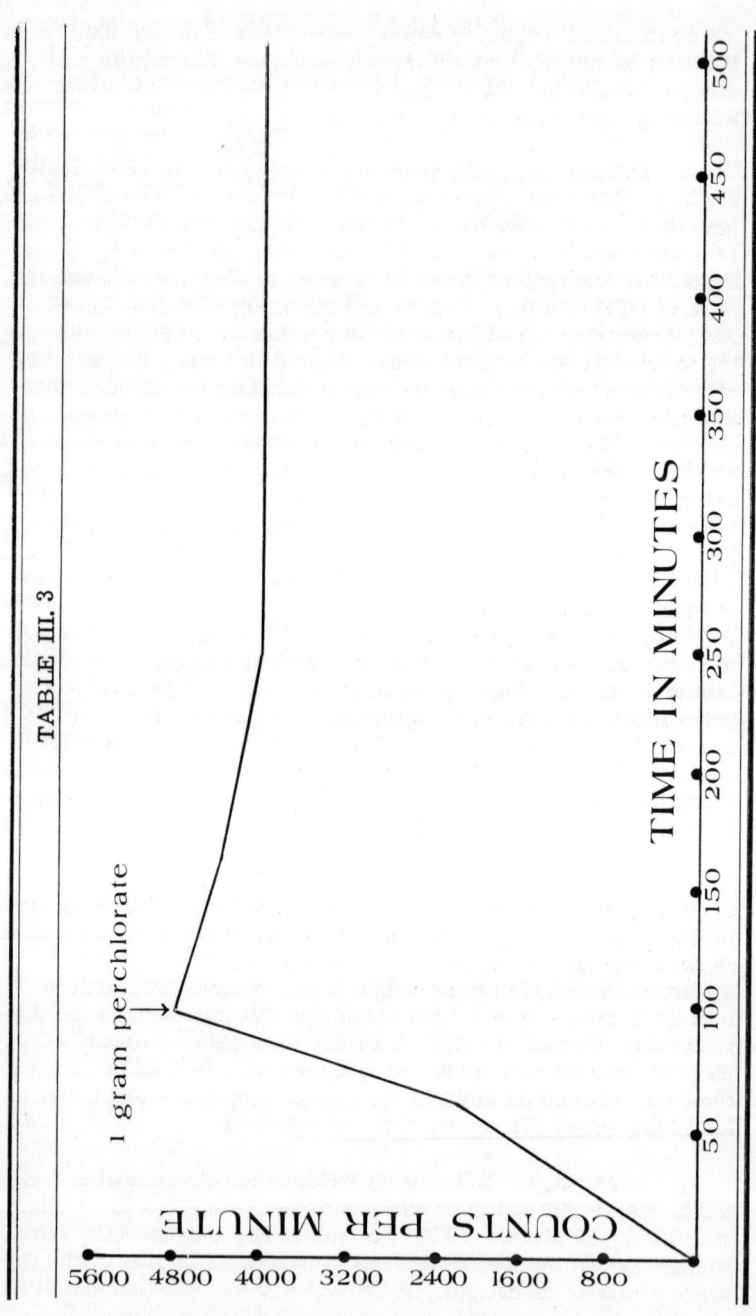

TABLE III. 3

mcgm%). The dose of the MMI was lowered to 10 mg every 12 hours. One month later the T4 was 2.5 mcgm% and the MMI was reduced to 2.5 mg every 12 hours. In the interval between April and September the patient remained euthyroid on the same dose of MMI. When therapy was discontinued in October a T4 was 7.1 mcgm%. The hyperthyroidism has remained in remission. A T4 in December, 1978, was 11.3 mcgm% (normal 4-12 mcgm%).

The case illustrates that permanent remission still occurs with a course of MMI. The improvement appeared within the first few weeks of therapy and was complete by three months. As is often the case appearance of hypothyroidism required reduction of the dose of MMI. Careful observation of the T4 will prevent the appearance of the symptoms of hypothyroidism. Once this happens either the dose of the thioamide must be reduced or a thyroid supplement added. The easiest solution is to reduce the dose of MMI or PTU to maintain euthyroidism. When the thyroid enlarges on therapy it will sometimes be necessary to add thyroid supplement. As thyroid function is reduced the normal pituitary-thyroid mechanism comes into play and through TSH stimulates the thyroid to produce more of its hormones and cause enlargement of the thyroid. A minimal dose of MMI controlled the patient for most of the duration of the therapy. All of the usual factors outlined previously were present to herald a permanent remission. MMI was selected because of the patient's wishes to avoid surgery if at all possible and since ablation with ^{131}I was declined. In this circumstance a short course of MMI would not have been indicated. The inconvenience to the patient was minimal and the response to therapy most rewarding.

The flow diagram in Figure 3.2 summarizes the use of PTU or MMI as definitive therapy. As long as the physician and the patient understand the shortcomings of the use of a thioamide this modality still has some justification.

38/ Drug Therapy of Hyperthyroidism

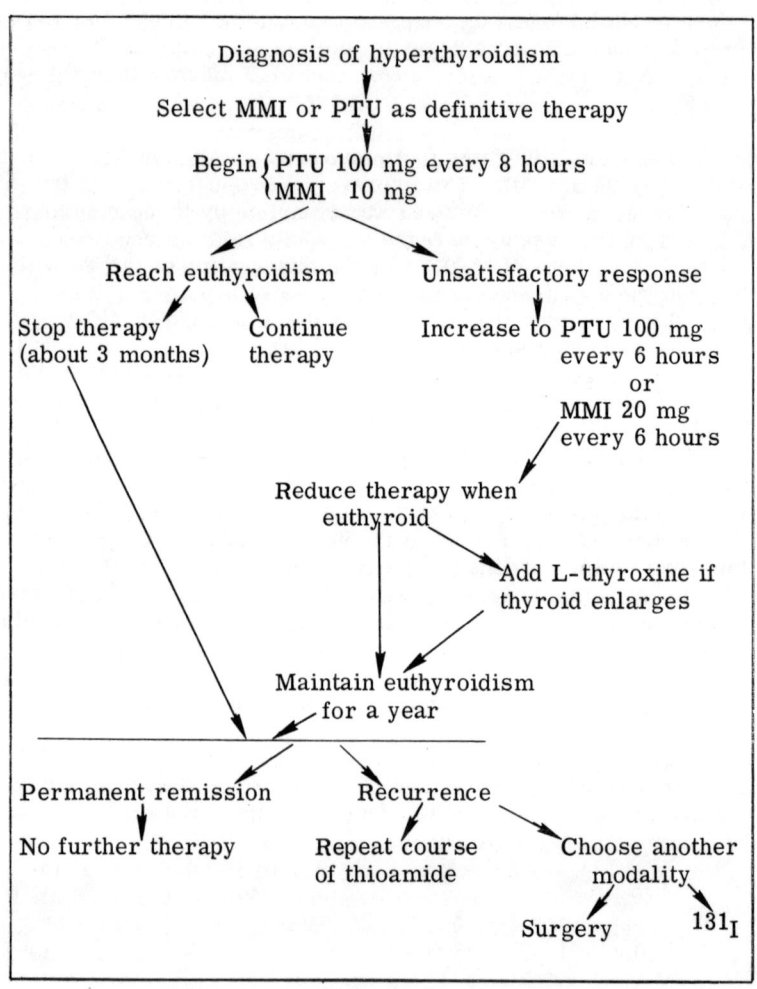

FIGURE 3.2: PTU OR MMI THERAPY

REFERENCES

1. Barzilai, D, Sheinfeld, J: Fatal complications following use of potassium perchlorate in thyrotoxicosis. Report of two cases and a review of the literature. Isr J Med Sci 2:453, 1966.

2. Reveno, WS, Rosenbaum, H: Observations on the use of antithyroid drugs. Ann Intern Med 60:980, 1964.

3. Wilcox, PH: Twelve years' experience of antithyroid treatment. Post grad Med J 38:275, 1962.

4. Hershman, JM: The treatment of hyperthyroidism. Ann Intern Med 64:1306, 1966.

5. Wartofsky, L: Low remission after therapy for Graves' Disease. JAMA 226:1083, 1973.

5a Shizume, K, Irie, M, Nagataki, S: Long-term result of antithyroid drug therapy for Graves' Disease: Follow up after more than 5 years. Endocrinologia Japonica 17:327, 1970.

6. Alexander, WD, Harden, RM, Koutras, DA, Wayne, E: Influence of iodine intake after treatment with antithyroid drugs. Lancet 2:866, 1965.

7. Lumholtz, IB, Poulsen, DL, Siersboek-Nielson, D, et al.: Outcome of long-term antithyroid treatment of Graves' Disease in relation to iodine intake. Acta Endocrinol. 84:538, 1977.

8. Wilson, GM: The treatment of thyrotoxicosis, In Symposium - Thyroid Disease and Calcium Metabolism, Edinburgh, 1966. The Royal College of Physicians of Edinburgh, 1967, pp. 51. (Royal College of Physicians of Edinburgh publication no. 33).

9. Greer, MA, Meihoff, WC, Stude, H: Treatment of hyperthyroidism with a single daily dose of propylthiouracil. N Engl J Med 272:888, 1965.

10. Hershman, JM, Givens, Jr, Cassidy, CE, Astwood, EB: Long-term outcome of hyperthyroidism treated with antithyroid drugs. J Clin Endocrinol Metab 26:803, 1966.

11. Irvine, WJ, Gray, RS, Morris, PJ, et al.: Correlation of HLA and thyroid antibodies with clinical course of thyrotoxicosis treated with antithyroid drugs. Lancet 2:898, 1977.

12. Sitar, DS, Abu-Bakare, A, Gardiner, RJ, et al.: Effect of chronic administration of propylthiouracil on its disposition during the treatment of hyperthyroidism. Thyroid Research; Proceedings of the Seventh International Thyroid Conference, Boston, June 9-13, 1975. Edited by Jacob Robbins. Amsterdam, Excerpta Medica, 1976, p. 425 (International congress series, no. 378).

13. Vesell, ES, Shapiro, Jr, Passananti, GT, et al.: Altered plasma half-lives of antipyrine, propylthiouracil, and methimazole in thyroid dysfunction. Clin Pharmacol Ther 17:48, 1975.

14. Sitar, DS, Hunningbake, DB: Pharmacokinetics of propylthyiouracil in man after a single oral dose. J Clin Endocrinol Metab 40:26, 1975.

15. Alexander, WD, Harden, RM, Shimmins, J: Thyroidal suppression by triiodothyronine as a guide to duration of treatment of thyrotoxicosis with antithyroid drugs. Lancet 2:1041, 1966.

16. Gwinup, G: Prospective randomized comparison of propylthiouracil. JAMA 239:2457, 1978.

17. Greer, MA, Kammer, H, Bouma, DJ: Short-term antithyroid drug therapy for the thyrotoxicosis of Graves' disease. N Engl J Med 297:173, 1977.

18. Alexander, WD, McLarty, DG, Robertson, J, et al.: Prediction of long-term results of antithyroid drug therapy for thyrotoxicosis. J Clin Endocrinol Metab 30:540, 1970.

19. Solomon, DH, Beck, JC, Vanderlaan, WP: Prognosis of hyperthyroidism treated by antithyroid drugs. JAMA 152:201, 1953.

20. Iino, S, Yamada, T, Greer, MA: Effect of graded doses of prophylthiouracil on biosynthesis of thyroid hormones. Endocrinology 68:582, 1961.

21. Richards, JB, Ingbar, SH: The effects of propylthiouracil and perchlorate on the biogenesis of thyroid hormone. Endocrinology 65:198, 1959.

22. Nagataki, S, Uchimura, H, Matsuzaki, F, Masuyama, Y: Comparison of the triiodothyronine suppression test by the twenty-minute and twenty-four-hour thyroidal ^{131}I uptake in patients receiving thioamide drugs. J Clin Endocrinol Metab 38:255, 1974.

23. Papapetrou, PD, Mothon, S, Alexander, WD: Binding of the ^{35}S of ^{35}S-propylthiouracil by follicular thyroglobulin in vino and in vitro.

24. Hosoya, T: Effect of various reagents including antithyroid compounds upon the activity of thyroid peroxidase. J Biochem 53:381, 1963.

25. Morris, DR, Hager, LP: Mechanism of the inhibition of enzymatic halogination by antithyroid agents. J Biol Chem 241:3582, 1966.

26. Taurog, A: The mechanism of action of the thioureylene drugs. Endocrinology 98:1031, 1976.

26a Nakashima, T, Taurog, A, Riesco, G: Mechanism of the action of thioureylene antithyroid drugs: Factors affecting intrathyroid metabolism of propylthiouracil and methimazole in rats. Endocrinology 103:2187, 1978.

27. Oppenheimer, JH, Schwarta, HL, Surks, MI: Propylthiouracil inhibits the conversion of L-thyroxine to L-triiodothyronine. J Clin Invest 51:2493, 1972.

28. Saberi, M, Sterling, FH, Utiger, RD: Reduction in extrathyroidal triiodothyronine production by propylthiouracil in man. J Clin Invest 55:218, 1975.

29. Geffner, DL, Azukizawa, M, Hershman, JM: Propylthiouracil blocks extrathyroidal conversion of thyroxine to triiodothyronine and augments thyrotropin secretion in man. J Clin Invest 55:224, 1975.

30. Vanderlaan, WP, Storie, VM: A survery of the factors controlling thyroid function, with special reference to newer views on antithyroid substances. Pharmacol Rev 7:301, 1955.

31. Edell, SL, Bartuska, DG: Aplastic anemia secondary to methimazole-case report and review of hematologic side effects. J Am Med Wom Assoc 30:412, 1975.

32. McGavack, TH, Chevalley, J: Untoward hematologic responses to the antithyroid compounds. Am J Med 17:36, 1954.

33. Amrhein, JA, Kenny, FM, Ross, D: Granulacytopenia, lupus-like syndrome, and other complications of propylthiouracil therapy. J Pediatr 76:54, 1970.

34. Breese, TJ, Solomon, IL: Granulocytopenia and hemolytic anemia as complications of propylthiouracil therapy. J Pediatr 86:117, 1975.

35. McClellan, JE, Wallingford, WR: Case reports plastic anemia due to methimazole. Va Med Mon 103:354, 1976.

36. Martelo, OJ, Katims, RB, Yunis, AA: Bone marrow aplasia following propylthiouracil therapy. Arch Intern Med 120:587, 1967.

37. Farbman, K, Wheeler, MF, Glick, SM: Arthritis induced by antithyroid medication. NY State J Med 69:826, 1969.

38. Gilbert, DK: Hypoprothrombinemia as a complication of propylthiouracil. JAMA 189:855, 1964.

39. Gotta, AW, Sullivan, CA, Seaman, J, Jean-Gilles, B: Prolonged intraoperative bleeding caused by propylthiouracil induced hypoprothrombinemia. Anesthesiology 37: 562, 1972.

40. Fischer, MG, Noyer, HR, Miller, A: Methimazole-induced jaundice. JAMA 223:1028, 1973.

41. Hung, W, August, GP: A "collagen-like" syndrome associated with antithyroid therapy. J Pediatr 82:852, 1973.

42. Wiberg, JJ, Nuttall, FQ: Methimazole toxicity from high doses. Ann Intern Med 77:414, 1972.

43. Berson, SA, Yalow, RS: Quantitative aspects of iodine metabolism. J Clin Invest 33:1533, 1954.

44. Abuid, J, Larsen, PR: Triodothyronine and thyroxine in hyperthyroidism. J Clin Invest 54:201, 1974.

45. Mortimer, CH, Anderson, DC, Liendo-CH, P, et al.: Thyrotoxicosis: relations between clinical state and biochemical changes during carbimazole treatment. Br Med J 1:138, 1977.

46. Jaffiol, C, Baldet, L, Khalil, R: Confrontation de deux techniques d'etude du test au thiocyanate de potassium. Applications cliniques. Ann Endocrinol 30:447, 1969.

47. Tamai, H, Nakagawa, T, Fukino, O: Thionamide Therapy in Graves' Disease: Relation of Relapse Rate to Duration of Therapy. Ann Intern Med 92:488, 1980.

PART TWO: DRUGS OTHER THAN THIOAMIDES

Agents as guanethidine, reserpine, propranolol, iodine, phenobarbital, and lithium have been used to reduce the clinical manifestations of hyperthyroidism. Unlike propylthiouracil (PTU) or methimazole (MMI) the improvement appears relatively rapidly and persists only as long as the agent is continued. In other words, permanent remission does not follow as it does with a course of one of the thioamides. The adrenergic blocking agents are effective in spite of the fact that most of the manifestations of hyperthyroidism probably stem from a direct peripheral action of the thyroid hormones rather than through an action of the sympathetic nervous system.[1,2] To achieve control of the symptoms and signs of hyperthyroidism propranolol has supplanted the other available agents. The role of iodine in the preoperative preparation for subtotal thyroidectomy is discussed in Chapter IV. Table III. 4 outlines the use of these agents.

There are many circumstances in the course of hyperthyroidism to consider rapid control of clinical manifestations. Often when diagnostic studies require a delay between the confirmation of the diagnosis of hyperthyroidism and the selection of a modality of definitive therapy, the patients can be made more comfortable with propranolol. This drug does not affect all of the parameters of thyroid function and thus will not interfere with the confirmation of the diagnosis. Or once the diagnosis is made and a patient is started on either MMI or PTU, at least six weeks are required before euthyroidism is reached. Here again propranolol can produce rapid relief from the symptoms of hyperthyroidism far more rapidly and lessen the discomfort from these symptoms. If ^{131}I ablation is selected for definitive therapy then it is necessary to wait at least three months before judging the effectiveness of a therapeutic dose of the isotope. Symptomatic control can be achieved with a thioamide or propranolol. The severity of the hyperthyroidism will determine whether or not symptomatic control is required and how rapidly it must be obtained. Finally survival in thyroid storm has improved remarkably with the use of a combination of these agents.

GUANETHIDINE

Guanethidine was one of the first adrenergic blocking agents tried in the control of the symptoms of hyperthyroidism, and was of

TABLE III.4

Agent	Route	Average Dose	Onset	Disadvantages
Guane-thidine	oral	50-75 mg (single daily dose)	3-5 days	Significant postural hypotension
Reserpine	oral	0.25 mg every 6 hours	2-4 weeks (full effect)	Somnolence gastrointestinal bleeding depression
	intra-muscular	2-4 mg every 4-6 hours	6-8 hours	
Pro-pranolol	oral	40 mg every 6 hours	1-2 days	Congestive heart failure
	intra-venous	1-2 mg every 4-6 hours	minutes	Asthma
Iodide	intra-venous	1 gram KI slowly over 8 hours	hours	increases iodine pool
	oral	2-3 drops Lugol's solution in juice T10		Escape after 2 weeks
Pheno-barbital	oral	15 mg every 6 hours		Sedation

limited usefulness. The drug can only be administered orally, requires at least three to five days for its full effect to appear and almost always produces significant postural hypotension.[3] It does not effect the thyroid and will not alter thyroid function tests.

RESERPINE

Although supplanted in most circumstances by propranolol, reserpine is still used in the treatment of thyroid storm.[4] A response will occur within 6-8 hours after an intramuscular dose. It is usually wise to begin with 1 mg and then depending on the response repeat the dose at 4-6 hour intervals or increase the size of the dose or decrease the interval between doses until a maximum of 4 mg every 4 hours is reached. In this way it will be possible to use the smallest dose to yield the greatest effect. On the other hand when reserpine is given orally a full effect will not appear until 2-4 weeks following the start of the medication. Most patients will respond to 0.25 mg given every 6 hours. The dose can then be reduced as necessary to maintain control of the symptoms. Side-effects of reserpine include excessive somnolence, gastrointestinal bleeding, depression, and on rare occasions, the carcinoid syndrome.[5] Needless to say the production of somnolence may be helpful in the agitated patient in thyroid storm. The greatest drawback to the use of reserpine is the relatively long delay before improvement occurs even when the intramuscular route is employed.

PROPRANOLOL

Propranolol quickly gained acceptance as an agent for the control of the symptoms of hyperthyroidism. It has many advantages over reserpine and guanethidine. These include the rapidity and reliability with which improvement occurs, the safety of the drug, and the availability of both an oral and an intravenous preparation. As effective as the drug is for the control of the symptoms of hyperthyroidism, it should not be used as the sole means of managing the disease. Symptoms improve dramatically but many of the adverse effects of hyperthyroidism are not reversed.[6] Thus the increased myocardial contractility of hyperthyroidism does not return to normal, and the depletion of fat and protein of the untreated disease is not corrected after long term use of propranolol. Thus it cannot substitute for either MMI or PTU as a drug for the definitive therapy of hyperthyroidism. In spite of the overall improvement seen with the medication, eye signs remain unchanged even if a propranolol solution is instilled directly into the eyes.[7,8]

Drug Therapy of Hyperthyroidism /47

Several other less common complications do respond to propranolol. The proximal myopathy of hyperthyroidism can be quite incapacitating and the drug has proven quite successful in the treatment of this problem.[9,10] Weakness often improves in a matter of days to allow ambulation to begin for an otherwise bed ridden patient. Another use of propranolol is in the treatment of symptomatic hypercalcemia in hyperthyroidism.[11] Although calcium is unaffected by propranolol in the hyperthyroid patient without hypercalcemia, elevated levels will fall during an infusion of propranolol or during the oral administration of the drug. This response to oral propranolol will occur within a day or so but does require titration of the dose to lower calcium.

There are certain limitations to the use of propranolol in the hyperthyroid patient. It should not be used in patients with congestive failure or asthma. Both will usually become worse on the drug. Propranolol should only be used for short term control of symptoms in pregnancy. There is evidence that it stimulates uterine muscle and may produce a small placenta and in turn retard fetal growth.[12] There is also the risk of depression of the fetus at term as well as those of bradycardia and hypoglycemia. Propranolol does permit control of the hyperthyroidism during pregnancy so that a decision about definitive therapy can be made when fetal safety is not a consideration. Yet the merits[13] of this approach do not seem very strong in the face of the question of the adverse effects of propranolol during pregnancy and the fact that all of the manifestations of hyperthyroidism are not reversed by it. Finally it must be kept in mind that an adequate block of the symptoms of hyperthyroidism with propranolol may not prevent the occurrence of thyroid storm.[14]

In the more urgent situations propranolol may be given intravenously as a dose of 1-2 mg using the fall in pulse rate as a guide to therapy. The dose is repeated every 4-6 hours as required to maintain the desired pulse rate. As soon as possible an oral dose of 20-40 mg can be substituted at 6-hour intervals. In less urgent situations the initial oral dose of propranolol is usually 10 mg every 6 hours. Since the response is seen within 24 hours it is possible to increase the dose when necessary at this interval until the desired level of control is achieved. A good guideline is to reduce the pulse to below 90/minute at rest. Considering the brief duration of action it is prudent to taper propranolol slowly rather than stopping the drug suddenly. This should avoid any flare of symptoms. Ordinarily a dose of 20-40 mg every 6 hours will be adequate to control symptoms.

One of the advantages of the adrenergic blocking agents as guanethidine or reserpine is that thyroid function tests are not altered. This would follow since the mechanism of action of these drugs is through an extrathyroidal, peripheral effect. The use of propranolol requires some qualification. Unlike these other two agents propranolol reduces the peripheral conversion of T4 to T3. There is in addition a rise in the ratio of reverse-T3 to T4.[14] Although values for T3 do not fall into the normal range, this effect should be kept in mind when evaluating the results of a T3 determination in a hyperthyroid patient on propranolol. Furthermore, this effect may provide an explanation for the mechanism by which propranolol controls the symptoms of hyperthyroidism. Rather than block the sympathetic nervous system perhaps propranolol by interfering with the metabolism of the thyroid hormones reduces their action on the cell. Or perhaps like the thioamides the final effect is a summation of many different mechanisms which depend on the degree of hyperthyroidism, as well as the route and concentration of propranolol.

IODINE

Iodine is used to prepare patients for subtotal thyroidectomy, and to treat thyroid storm. It has been added to a course of MMI or PTU in an attempt to increase the rate of permanent remissions, and has also been used following a dose of ^{131}I to control the symptoms of hyperthyroidism until the full effect of radioiodine appears. The treatment of thyroid storm is covered in Chapter VII. Since with MMI or PTU the thyroid becomes quite vascular, iodine is added to the preparation 10-14 days before surgery to reduce this effect. When propranolol is used to prepare for thyroid surgery this effect does not appear and therefore iodine is probably unnecessary. For preoperative preparation, the dose of iodine is 2 or 3 drops of Lugol's Solution 3 times daily in juice. The merits of the use of iodine after ^{131}I ablation are discussed in Chapter VI.

There are many limitations to the use of iodine in hyperthyroidism. Both symptoms and thyroid function tests improve rapidly during the first week of iodine therapy, but the effect usually will not persist beyond the second week of therapy since escape rapidly occurs.[16] Another drawback is that large doses of exogenous iodine flood the extrathyroidal iodine pool and thus prevent measurements of thyroid iodine uptake with a radioactive isotope or for that matter interfere with radioiodine ablation. This large extrathyroidal iodine pool raises the risk of increasing the supply of iodide to the thyroid should the block with MMI or PTU be insufficient. The net result can be an exacerbation of the hyperthyroidism. Early accounts of the use of thioamides failed to support this contention[18] so that the risk is undoubtedly more theoretical than real. The thyroid is quite sensitive to iodide following surgery or ^{131}I ablation, so that in either case hypothyroidism may appear quite rapidly.[20] It is reversible but its appearance can certainly complicate rather than simplify the course of therapy.[19] It is actually easier to control the hyperthyroidism with MMI or PTU alone and await recurrence either after a brief 3-month course or a more prolonged one-year course. In radioiodine ablation controlling the symptoms with PTU or MMI or even propranolol provides a far more satisfactory means to control the symptoms while awaiting the permanent effects of the isotope.

The mechanisms through which iodine brings about its effects differs somewhat according to the circumstances in which it is used. In thyroid storm it blocks the release of T3 and T4 from the thyroid.[21] The effect appears within a 8-hour period and by preventing entry of the hormones into the extrathyroidal pool, allows that pool to diminish rapidly in size. Iodine does not influence the conversion of T4 to T3 or subsequent metabolism.[22] The response of the thyroid to iodine in preparation for thyroid surgery is discussed in Chapter V. The mechanism of action with prolonged use remains unclear.[23] Hormonal synthesis is blocked with iodide in acute experiments but this may not be the mechanism with more chronic use.

In summary then iodide is still used in preparing the patient for subtotal thyroidectomy and in treating thyroid storm. For the control of the symptoms of hyperthyroidism it has been supplanted by propranolol.

LITHIUM

The use of lithium in the treatment of hyperthyroidism stems from the observation that goiters appeared in patients receiving lithium for psychiatric illnesses.[24] In clinical trials lithium controlled the symptoms of hyperthyroidism for as long as 6 months, but showed no advantage when compared to a thioamide as MMI.[26] Furthermore there are frequent, incapacitating side effects even with relatively low doses of lithium and relapse occurs quite rapidly once the drug is stopped. The mechanism of action involves the inhibition of the release of the thyroid hormones and a more rapid disappearance of T4. The failure to block the accumulation of T3 and T4 within the thyroid raises the problem of exacerbation whenever release of these hormones occurs. It is best to consider lithium as an agent to control the symptoms of hyperthyroidism only when all the other agents have either failed or produced serious complications.[28]

PHENOBARBITAL

Phenobarbital is usually added because of its sedative effect. However, its beneficial effect may also derive in part from its influence on the metabolic clearance of T4.[29]

REFERENCES

1. Levey, GS: Catecholamine Sensitivity, thyroid hormone and the heart. Amer J Med 50:413, 1971.

2. Zivillich, CW, Matthay, M, Potts, DE, et al.: Thyrotoxicosis: Comparison of effects of thyroid ablation and beta-adrenergic blockage on metabolic rate and ventilatory control. J Clin Endocrinol Metab 46:491, 1978.

3. Lee, WY, Bronsky, D, Waldstein, SS: Studies of thyroid and sympathetic nervous system interrelationships. II. Effects of guanethidine on manifestations of hyperthyroidism. J Clin Endocrinol Metab 22:879, 1962.

4. Canary, JJ, Schaaf, M, Duffy, BJ Jr, et al.: Effects of oral and intramuscular administration of reserpine in thyrotoxicosis. N Engl J Med 257:435, 1957.

5. Blumenthal, M, Danes, R, Dee, R: Carcinoid syndrome following reserpine therapy in thyrotoxicosis. Arch Intern Med 116:819, 1965.

6. Mazzaferri, EL, Reynolds, JC, Young, RL, et al.: Propranolol as primary therapy for thyrotoxicosis. Arch Intern Med 136:50, 1976.

7. Sneddon, JM, Turner, P: Adrenergic blockade and the eye signs of thyrotoxicosis. Lancet 2:525, 1966.

8. Murchison, LE, Bewsher, PD, Chesters, MI, Ferrer, WR: Comparison of propranolol and practolol in the management of hyperthyroidism. Br J Clin Pharmacol 3:273, 1976.

9. Pimstone, D, Marine, N, Pimstone, B: Beta-adrenergic blockade in thyrotoxic myopathy. Lancet 2:1219, 1968.

10. Rothberg, MP, Shebert, RT, Levey, GS, Daroff, RB: Propranolol and hyperthyroidism. Reversal of upper motor neuron signs. JAMA 230:1017, 1974.

11. Rude, RK, Oldham, SB, Singer, FR, Nicoloff, Jr: Treatment of thyrotoxic hypercalcemia with propranolol. N Engl J Med 294:431, 1976.

12. Bullock, JL, Harris, RE, Young, R: Treatment of thyrotoxicosis during pregnancy with propranolol. Am J Obstet-Gynecol 121:242, 1975.

13. Gladstone, GR, Hordof, A, Gersony, WM: Propranolol administration during pregnancy: Effects on the fetus J Pediatr 86:962, 1975.

14. Eriksson, M, Rubenfeld, S, Garber, AJ, Kohler, P.O.: Propranolol does not prevent thyroid storm. N Engl J Med 296:263, 1977.

15. Verhoeven, RP, Visser, TJ, Docter, R, et al.: Plasma thyroxine, 3, 3', 5-triiodothyronine and 3, 3', 5-triiodothyronine during b-adrenergic blockade in hyperthyroidism. J Clin Endocrinol Metab 44:1002, 1977.

16. Emerson, CH, Anderson, AJ, Howard, WJ, Utiger, RD: Serum thyroxine and triiodothyronine concentrations during iodide treatment of hyperthyroidism. J Clin Endocrinol Metab 40:33, 1975.

17. Croxson, MS, Hall, TD, Nicoloff, JT: Combination drug therapy for treatment of hyperthyroid Graves' disease. J Clin Endocrinol Metab 45:623, 1977.

18. Winkler, AW, Man, EB, Danowski, TS: Minimum dosage of thiourea, given together with iodine medication, necessary for the production and maintenance of a remission in hyperthyroidism. J Clin Invest 26:446, 1947.

19. Hagen, GA, Ouellette, RP, Chapman, EM: Comparison of high and low dosage levels of ^{131}I in the treatment of thyrotoxicosis. N Engl J Med 277:559, 1967.

20. Braverman, LE, Woeber, KA, Ingbar, SH: Induction of myxedema by iodide in patients euthyroid after radioiodine or surgical treatment of diffuse toxic goiter. N Engl J Med 281:816, 1969.

21. Wartofsky, L, Ransil, BJ, Ingbar, SH: Inhibition by iodine of the release of thyroxine from the thyroid glands of patients with thyrotoxicosis. J Clin Invest 49:78, 1970.

22. Wolff, J: Iodide goiter and the pharmacologic effects of excess iodide. Am J Med 47:101, 1969.

23. Degroot, LJ: Action of potassium iodide on thyroxine metabolism. J Clin Endocrinol Metab 26:778, 1966.

24. Schou, M, Admisen, A, Jensen, SE, Olsen, T: Occurrence of goiter during lithium treatment. Brit Med J 3:710, 1968.

25. Lazarus, JH, Addison, GM, Richards, AR, Owen, GM: Treatment of thyrotoxicosis with lithium carbonate. Lancet 2:1160, 1974.

26. Kristensen, O, Andersen, HH, Pallisgaard, G: Lithium carbonate in the treatment of thyrotoxicosis. A controlled trial. Lancet 1:603, 1976.

27. Temple, R, Berman, M, Robbins, Jr, Wolff, J: The use of lithium in the treatment of thyrotoxicosis. J Clin Invest 51:2746, 1972.

28. Eulry, F, Orgiozzi, J, Mornex, R: Les sels de lithium ont-ils leur place dans le traitement des hyperthyroidies graves? Nouv Presse Med 6:2955, 1977.

29. Hufner, M, Knopfle, M: Pharmacological influences on T4 and T3 conversion in rats. Clin Chim Acta 72:337, 1976.

CHAPTER IV

SURGERY AND HYPERTHYROIDISM

It is always tempting for the internist to minimize the indications for any surgical procedure. So often this approach occurs in the consideration of subtotal thyroidectomy for the treatment of hyperthyroidism. Yet as one of the choices for definitive therapy, it remains as important as the thioamides or ^{131}I ablation. Reservations about its usefulness include considerations related to the thyroid itself--recurrence of the hyperthyroidism, and the appearance of hypothyroidism, damage to nearby structures--production of hypocalcemia, damage to the recurrent and external laryngeal nerves, and finally those related to surgical technique--mortality from the procedure, uncontrolled bleeding, and scar formation. There is no question that one striking advantage for surgery is the relative rapidity with which cure of the hyperthyroidism can be accomplished. Adding the time required for preparing the patient for surgery to the time required for hospitalization for the surgery plus the interval for postoperative convalescence, the total duration will usually be less than three months. Preoperative preparation with propranolol will reduce the total period to less than six weeks. This compares with a minimum of three months to judge the effectiveness of a single dose of ^{131}I or from 6-18 months to decide whether a course of a thioamide will produce a permanent remission.

HYPOTHYROIDISM AND RECURRENCE OF HYPERTHYROIDISM

In the hands of experienced thyroid surgeons the incidence of hyperthyroidism varies from as low as 3%[1] to as high as 9%.[2] Even the higher rate of recurrence compares favorably with a course of a thioamide in which the incidence of permanent remission is only 30%. The incidence of hypothyroidism following surgery may be as high as 48%.[1] Comparison with radioiodine is not appropriate with regard to recurrences since once repeated doses of the isotope are taken into account all patients will respond. However, the occurrence of hypothyroidism is far higher following radioiodine. Hypothyroidism that appears during the course of a thioamide will disappear once the drug is stopped.

One might view the appearance of hypothyroidism and the recurrence of hyperthyroidism in terms of the size of the thyroid remnant following surgery. Attempts to reduce the rate of recurrence by decreasing the amount of thyroid left tend to increase the incidence of hypothyroidism. For example, leaving only 2-4 grams of thyroid will yield an incidence of hypothyroidism of 66% but increasing the size of the remnant to more than 10 grams still produces hypothyroidism in 21% of the patients.[3] With comparable ranges of thyroid remnants recurrence occurs in 15% of patients with large remnants and 2.1% of patients with the smaller remnants.[4] There is however little relationship between the size of the gland before surgery and the subsequent development of hypothyroidism. Hence the conclusion is that once the problems of risks of hypothyroidism and the recurrence of hyperthyroidism are balanced, the occurrence of hypothyroidism is an inevitable consequence of subtotal thyroidectomy as it is following radioiodine.

Since autoimmunity is considered by some authorities in the pathogenesis of hyperthyroidism, this mechanism provides another explanation for the appearance of hypothyroidism following surgery. Unfortunately the correlation of antithyroid antibodies measured by several techniques and the appearance of hypothyroidism though high in some studies[5] is not statistically significant in others.[3,6] Another marker of autoimmunity is the presence of specific cellular infiltrates in the surgical specimen. The infiltration of lymphoid cells is greater in the thyroids of patients who are found to have antithyroid antibodies before surgery.[6,7] Yet predicting the development of hypothyroidism correlates better with the size of the thyroid remnant than with a specific cellular infiltrate. More over lymphocytic infiltration appears important in some studies[3] and plasma cell and lymphoid follicles in others.[7] The role of any of these parameters of autoimmunity in predicting the occurrence of hypothyroidism is too uncertain at present to be helpful.

Hypothyroidism usually appears within one or two years after surgery though there is some evidence that it may continue to appear indefinitely after surgery much as it does after radioiodine therapy.[8] In contrast the recurrence of hyperthyroidism may occur anytime after surgery and has been documented as long as 50 years afterward.[9] It is thus imperative that careful follow up be a matter of course after the surgery. Recurrence can be recognized by a recurrence of the symptoms and the presence of elevated thyroid function tests. Hypothyroidism presents more problems in the diagnosis. Thus levels of plasma thyrotropin (TSH) may be elevated following surgery but all patients with elevated levels of TSH do not become hypothyroid.[9] Values for triiodothyronine are often within the normal range regardless of whether the patient is euthyroid or hypothyroid.[10] Prolonged observation of patients considered hypothyroid brings up the possibility that in many the underactivity is only transient and that permanent thyroid replacement is not necessary.[11, 28] It seems wise therefore to maintain careful follow up of the patient after surgery, using the appearance of the signs and symptoms of hypothyroidism plus confirmation with measurement of plasma thyroxine to make a positive diagnosis. When the situation is equivocal it is quite prudent to continue follow up until the diagnosis is certain. The diagnosis of hypothyroidism commits the patient to life-long replacement and with a certain diagnosis future studies become unnecessary.

Once the diagnosis of hypothyroidism is certain replacement can be started with one of the preparations of L-thyroxine. A standard schedule is to begin with 0.05 mg every day and increase to full replacement by 0.05 mg increments every 2 weeks. The rapidity with which the dose is increased and the final dose reached will depend on the improvement of symptoms, correction of the abnormal thyroid function tests and the ability of the patient to tolerate replacement. The treatment of recurrence presents more problems. For most patients it will be necessary to use an ablative dose of radioiodine.[11a] This decision is often most difficult since radioiodine has usually been considered and eliminated when the initial choice of definitive therapy was made. The selection of surgery as the modality for treating these recurrences is not wise since most patients who have a recurrence and undergo a second thyroidectomy will have a second recurrence.[11b] Finally a course of one of the thioamides will only produce control of the hyperthyroidism during therapy but not remission once the course is completed.

OTHER COMPLICATIONS OF SURGERY

Table IV lists the more common complications of surgery. The best perspective to view operative mortality with adequate preoperative preparation is that in any one of a number of recent reviews the operative mortality was zero.[12] Certainly this should be the case in the hands of any experienced thyroid surgeon. The risks of thyroid storm should be obviated with the preoperative use of either propranolol or thioamide plus iodine. Adequate doses of propranolol, however, may not always prevent thyroid storm.[13] Damage to either the recurrent laryngeal nerve or the external laryngeal nerve are in part a function of surgical technique.[14,15] Many methods have been devised to avoid nerve damage.[16] Another form of nerve damage is Horner's Syndrome which occurs as a result of injury to the cervical sympathetic chain.[17] Complications as laryngeal edema and postoperative bleeding can usually be treated by careful observation. Rarely tracheostomy will be required.

Hypocalcemia is usually attributed to damage to the parathyroids during surgery and most commonly appears within the first twenty-four hours following surgery. The incidence of persistent hypocalcemia ranges between 1-2%,[18] however, transient hypocalcemia is far more common.[19] One objection to blaming parathyroid damge for all forms of hypocalcemia is that hypocalcemia occurs far less commonly following surgery on the thyroid when hyperthyroidism is not present.[20, 20a, 20b] Thus the transient hypocalcemia might occur because of bone involvement subsequent to hyperthyroidism.[19] Just as following parathyroid surgery for hyperparathyroidism, the so called "hungry bones" take up calcium once the disease process is reversed and very rapidly lower serum calcium. Once repletion of bone mineral is accomplished by repletion of calcium then serum calcium returns to normal. Permanent hypocalcemia reflects hypoparathyroidism.

Evidence for hypocalcemia may range from a positive Chvostek's or Trousseau's sign to tetany. Calcium values at the lower limits of normal, sometimes found in routing postoperative calciums, do not require therapy since more often than not this depression is only transient. With the appearance of symptoms or if values fall rapidly toward 6 mg% replacement

TABLE IV.1

COMPLICATIONS OF SURGERY

I Thyroid Related
   A) Recurrent hyperthyroidism
   B) Hypothyroidism
   C) Thyroid Storm

II Damage to Surrounding Structures
   A) Hypoparathyroidism
   B) Recurrent laryngeal nerve injury
   C) External laryngeal nerve injury
   D) Horner's Syndrome

III Miscellaneous
   A) Postoperative bleeding
   B) Laryngeal edema
   C) Excessive scar formation (Keloid)
   D) Surgical mortality and morbidity

with calcium is necessary. The first step is rapid intravenous infusion of calcium given as 10-20 cc of a 10% calcium gluconate solution. The infusion can be repeated very four to six hours as required. Or it can be infused slowly over an eight hour period, beginning with 40 ml of a 10% calcium gluconate solution. Response is judged by the improvement of symptoms and signs of hypocalcemia as well as by a rise in the serum calcium. The exact choice of the route and the form of calcium depend largely on experience. Once long term replacement is required it is easier to use an oral form of calcium. Response in this circumstance depends on administering about one gram of elemental calcium daily, a dose which becomes quite difficult using the intravenous route. For example a 10% solution of calcium contains only 100 mg of elemental calcium. The use of vitamin D preparations is reserved for permanent replacement in view of the long interval before an effect is seen and the long interval before such an effect is dissipated.

The following case illustrates the problems of replacement of calcium following surgery. The patient, a 27-year-old female underwent a subtotal thyroidectomy in March, 1977. The diagnosis of hyperthyroidism had been made in January and in the three month interval the patient had been prepared for surgery with propylthiouracil. Table IV.2 lists the postoperative calciums and the corresponding therapy for each day. The

TABLE IV.2

POSTOPERATIVE HYPOCALCEMIA

Day after surgery	Calcium (mg%)	Signs of Symptoms	Comment (Dose indicated per 24 hours)
0	8.7	0	Preoperative value
1	6.8	+	20 cc Ca Gluconate IV
2	6.4	+	30 cc Ca Gluconate IV
3	7.1	0	30 cc Ca Gluconate IV
4	5.9	+	Calcium lactate 4.3 g po and 90 cc Ca Gluconate IV
8	5.9	+	5.76 g Ca Lactate
11	5.5	+	Add Dihydrotachysterol (DHT) 1.2 mg
15	5.9	+	Increase DHT to 1.6 mg
20	7.7	0	

calcium dropped within the first 24 hours after surgery and the patient showed tetany. Intravenous calcium pushed the calcium to 7.1 mg%, however, this increase was not sustained and larger amounts of calcium given as oral calcium gluconate also failed to produce a response. Once it becomes clear that the hypocalcemia was not transient Dihydrotachysterol was added; however roughly 10 days elapsed before the calcium returned to a more satisfactory value. The difficulty in replacing calcium should be quite evident in this case.

SELECTION OF PATIENTS

The choice of subtotal thyroidectomy as the definitive therapy must balance several factors. It is indicated for patients in the age range of 20-40 who are not candidates for thioamides. Often it will be because the patient may fail to comply for the duration of therapy. The availability of propranolol for preoperative preparation allow such a patient to select surgery as a modality of therapy. It is indicated when speed is required between diagnosis and cure since as noted this modality achieves euthyroidism in the shortest interval of all modalities. It can be selected whenever a thioamide fails to produce a permanent remission. However in patients over 40 ablation with radioiodine presents a better alternative. Surgery is preferable in patients with a very large goiter since marked decrease in thyroid size does not reliably follow either radioiodine or thioamide therapy. The solitary overactive nodule is considered to be an indication for surgery by some authors.[21] However the merits of this indication must be weighed against the ease of administering radioiodine in these patients. Cancer of the thyroid is associated rarely with hyperthyroidism. When the configuration of the enlarged thyroid raises this consideration surgery will be required to resolve the dilemma. The following summarizes the indications for subtotal thyroidectomy:

1. Patients age 20-40
2. Failure for remission to occur with thioamide
3. Need for short course of therapy
4. Unreliable patients
5. Very large thyroids
6. Solitary nodules
7. Suspicion of thyroid carcinoma

PREPARATION OF PATIENTS

There are two methods used at present to prepare patients for surgery. Since thyroid storm may occur with any degree of hyperthyroidism, no matter how slight, it is important that subtotal thyroidectomy not be undertaken without adequate preparation. The more conventional, older approach is to render the patient clinically and chemically euthyroid with a thioamide as PTU or MMI. This requires 4-6 weeks to achieve. One week before surgery iodide is added to reduce the vascularity of the gland.

The use of iodide in preparing patients for surgery raises several questions. First, the usual explanation for the mechanism of action of iodide is that it produces involution of the gland and reduces vascularity. Careful histiometric observations suggest that a better explanation is that iodides cause an increase in the volume of colloid and this by compression reduces vascularity.[22] Secondly there is some uncertainty about the length of time that iodide preparation is required and the maximum time for which the effect will persist. Judging from older experience using iodide to control the symptoms of hyperthyroidism the minimum preparation should be no less than one week.[23] The maximum duration of therapy must be less than 3 weeks since thereafter escape will rapidly occur in most patients. Finally there is the question of the dose of iodide necessary to produce a satisfactory effect. Though a wide range has been employed, as little as 10 mg of elemental iodide has sufficed.[24] A safe approximation is to use 2 drops of Lugol's Solution three times daily for 7-10 days.[25] This will provide 50 mg of elemental iodide daily. Figure 4.1 lists some pertinent facts about Lugol's Solution and a saturated solution of potassium iodide.

Iodine Preparation	mg Iodine per ml
Lugol's Solution	125
Saturated solution of Potassium Iodide (SS KI)	760
1 drop SS KI = 6 drops Lugol's Solution = 50 mg Iodide	

FIGURE 4.1: Iodine Therapy

An alternate method is to prepare the patient with propranolol alone or in combination with iodide.[26,27] Since thyroid storm has occurred in hyperthyroid patients fully blocked with propranolol,[13] it is wise to limit this method to patients who cannot be prepared with a thioamide and iodide. The patient who has taken a thioamide eratically for a prolonged period before surgery will require iodide to produce involution. Otherwise iodide can safely be omitted from the preparation. Propranolol is started at 10 mg every six hours and titrated upward to reduce the resting pulse rate to less than 90/minute. As an inpatient these increases can be made at daily intervals. For the outpatient it is advisable to wait 3-4 days before increasing the dose. As an extra margin of safety it is wise to aim to reduce the pulse rate after brief exercise such as a brisk, short walk. Lowering the pulse after exercise to below 100-110/minute insures a full measure of block with propranolol. Most patients in the hospital can be prepared by this technique in about one week. Outpatient preparation will take somewhat longer. It is necessary to continue propranolol at the 6-hour interval until the surgery begins. After surgery and until the administration of the oral preoperative dose is possible, it will be necessary to continue the propranolol as an intravenous dose of 1-2 mg every 4-6 hours to keep the pulse below 90-100/minute. The flow diagram in Figure 4.2 outlines the preparation for surgery.

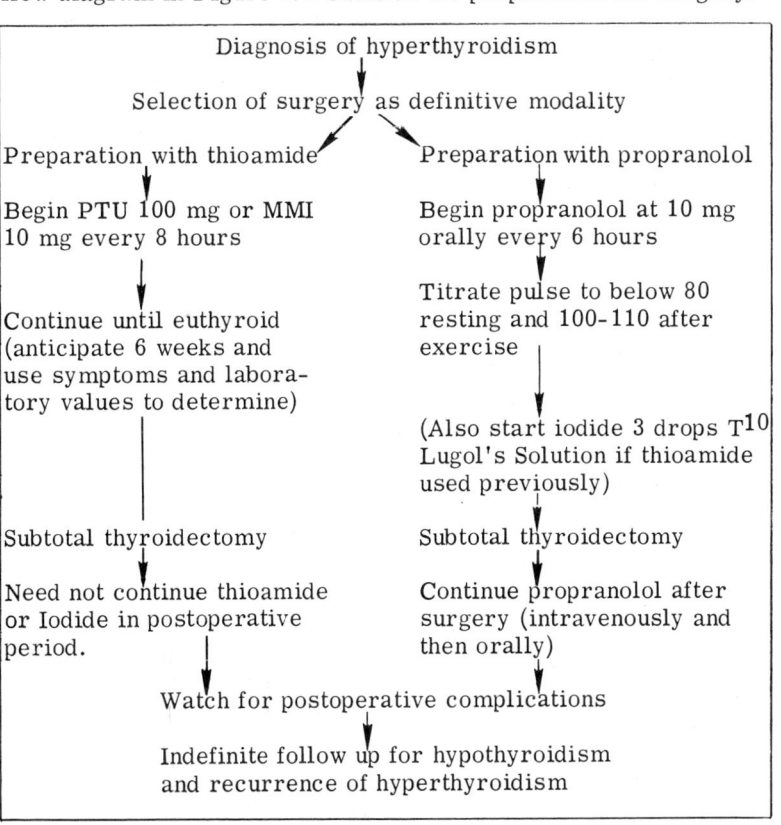

FIGURE 4.2: Flow Diagram For Preparation For Surgery

Surgery and Hyperthyroidism

The following cases will illustrate the selection of subtotal thyroidectomy for the treatment of hyperthyroidism and the methods for preparing the patients for surgery.

In the following case propranolol was used for preparation. The patient, a 24-year-old female was admitted to the hospital in February, 1978 for subtotal thyroidectomy. Her complaints which began one year previously included nervousness, weakness, irritability, weight loss, extreme fatigue and swelling of the neck. She had been treated with 6 miC of ^{131}I at another hospital September, 1977; however, there was no improvement in her symptoms. Following admission an attempt was made to prepare the patient for surgery with propranolol but the pulse failed to fall below 110/minute at rest even with 80 mg of the drug every 6 hours.

The patient was discharged from the hospital and placed on PTU 100 mg every 8 hours. In the interval from February to June, 1978, all symptoms disappeared and arrangements were made for admission in July, 1978. The T4 fell from 20 mcg% in February to 7 mcg% in June. On admission in July the patient appeared restless, and complained of increased sweating and palpitations. Her pulse rate was 125/minute. A T4 was mcg% and a T3 resin 42% (Normal 25-35%). On close questioning the patient admitted to omitting the PTU once arrangements had been made for the admission for thyroidectomy.

Since the patient was not euthyroid a second attempt at preparation with propranolol was made. Over a 10-day period from admission, the dose of propranolol was increased at daily intervals until a dose of 80 mg every 6 hours was reached. The pulse at rest was 88/minute with this dose. With exercise it rose to 108/minute and returned to the baseline at 2 minutes. Surgery proceeded without difficulty. Her pulse was maintained below 100/minute with an intravenous dose of propranolol of 0.5 mg every six hours for the first two postoperative days. The dose of oral propranolol was then resumed and tapered over a two week period. In August, 1978, a T4 was 7.1 mcg%.

The patient, although only 24 years old and for most physicians a candidate for either a thioamide or surgery, was treated with ^{131}I first. Euthyroidism was not achieved and once the patient understood all of the ramifications of ^{131}I ablation, she declined a second dose. It should be emphasized that once ablation with radioiodine is selected it is customary to continue with this modality until euthyroidism is achieved. The failure to control the symptoms with propranolol during the first hospital admission probably stems from the overwhelming effect of the thyroid secretion. The degree of hyperthyroidism was far too severe to obtain sufficient control in a brief period. Control was achieved with several months of PTU yet the patient failed to comply with therapy in the brief interval between her last outpatient visit and the hospital admission for the subtotal thyroidectomy. At this point it would not have been realistic to attempt to repeat the course of PTU. The preparation with propranolol was then successful and surgery was possible within 10 days after admission. It was necessary to continue the propranolol after surgery. Iodine was also used in that week of preoperative preparation in view of the prolonged use of PTU before admission. The patient represented an ideal candidate for surgery, and though unreliable, was prepared for surgery under careful supervision. It would have been necessary otherwise to repeat the dose of radioiodine. She has remained euthyroid following surgery. However, because of the possibility of recurrence of hyperthyroidism continued follow up will be essential.

A second case illustrates a more conventional approach to thyroid surgery. The symptoms of hyperthyroidism for this 16-year-old woman began in January, 1977. Her symptoms included weight loss, extreme irritability, personality change, hair loss, palpitations, pruritis, and increased sweating. On PTU from June, 1977, when the diagnosis of hyperthyroidism was first made until January, 1978 her symptoms slowly improved. However, she still was aware of great irritability, palpitations and the weight loss persisted. In March, 1978, the thyroid was enlarged to four times normal and there was a bruit. There was bilateral exophthalmos. Pulse was 110/minute. The patient was unwilling to continue the thioamide indefinitely and thus preparations were made for surgery. The dose of PTU was increased to 100 mg every 6 hours. In the interval from March to July her weight increased ten pounds and her pulse fell to 80/minute. Just before admission for surgery the T4 was 9.1 mcg% (Normal 5-12 mcg%) and the T3 resin, 31.3% (Normal 25-35%). In the week before surgery the patient was placed on Lugol's Solution using 3 drops three times daily. The surgery proceeded uneventfully permitting discharge from the hospital within one week after admission. In November, 1978 her T4 was 8.8 mcg% and T3 resin 39.3%.

This patient was an ideal candidate for surgery. Although she had agreed to a course of PTU, she was unwilling to continue the therapy without an assurance that a permanent remission would follow. Certainly control of her hyperthyroidism had not been achieved after nearly nine months of PTU therapy. This did not help in assuring the patient about the possibilities of permanent remission. An effective dose of PTU was employed to prepare the patient and the course thereafter was uneventful. Once the patient and her family understood the problems of PTU therapy it became clear that surgery would have been the better choice. Again it should be emphasized that the patient probably failed to take the PTU regularly. The hardest decision was to select surgery and yet this proved far easier than her frustrating year on PTU. She has remained euthyroid postoperatively but careful and continued follow up will be necessary.

REFERENCES

1. Beahrs, OH, Sakulsky, SB: Surgical thyroidectomy in the management of exophthalmic goiter Arch Surg 96:512, 1968.

2. Blichert - Toft, M, Jorgensen, SJ, Hansen, JB, Ibsen, J, Watt-Boolsen, S, Christiansen, C: Long term observation of thyroid function after surgical treatment of thyrotoxicosis. Acta Chir Scand 143:221, 1977.

3. Michie, W, Pegg, CAS, Bewsher, PD: Prediction of hypothyroidism after partial thyroidectomy for thyrotoxicosis. Br Med J 1:13, 1972.

4. Crile, G Jr, McCullagh, EP: The treatment of hyperthyroidism. Ann Surg 134:19, 1954.

5. Green, M, Wislon, GM: Thyrotoxicosis treated by surgery or iodine-131. With special reference to development of hypothyroidism. Br Med J 1:1005, 1964.

6. Van Welsum, M, Feltkamp, TEW, De Vries, MJ, et al.: Hypothyroidism after thyroidectomy for Graves' Disease: A search for an explanation. Br Med J 4:755, 1974.

7. Young, RJ, Beck, JW, Michie, W: The predictive value of histometry of thyroid tissue in anticipating hypothyroidism for primary thyrotoxicosis. J Clin Path 28:94, 1975.

8. Nofal, MM, Beierwaltes, WH, Patno, ME: Treatment of hyperthyroidism with sodium iodide I131. JAMA 197:605, 1966.

9. Hamburger, JI: Recurrent hyperthyroidism after thyroidectomy. Arch Surg 111:91, 1976.

10. Evered, D, Young, ET, Tunbridge, WM, et al.: Thyroid function after subtotal thyroidectomy for hyperthyroidism. Br Med J 1:25, 1975.

11. Toft, AD: Temporary hypothyroidism after surgical treatment of thyrotoxicosis. Lancet 2:817, 1976.

11a. Kalk, WJ, Kantor, S, Durbach, D, et al.: Post-thyroidectomy thyrotoxicosis. Lancet 1:291, 1978.

11b. Hedley, AJ, Flemming, CJ, Chesters, MI, et al.: Surgical treatment of thyrotoxicosis. Br Med J 1:519, 1970.

12. Gillquist, J, Karlberg, B, Sjodahl, R, Tegler, L: Preoperative treatment of hyperthyroidism. Effect on primary postoperative complications. Acta Chir Scand 140:23, 1974.

13. Eriksson, M, Rubenfeld, A, Garber, AJ, Kohler, PO: Propranolol does not prevent thyroid storm. N Engl J Med 296:263, 1977.

14. Riddell, V: Thyroidectomy: Prevention of bilateral recurrent nerve palsy. Br J Surg 57:1, 1970.

15. Moosman, DA, Deweese, MS: The external laryngeal nerve as related to thyroidectomy. Surg Gynecol Obstet 127:1011, 1968.

16. Kratz, RC: Vocal cord paralysis and thyroid surgery. Annals Otology, Rhinology, Laryngology 87:383, 1978.

17. Smith, I, Murley, RS: Damage to the cervical sympathetic system during operations on the thyroid gland. Br J Surg 52:673, 1965.

18. McNeill, AD, Thomson, JA: Long-term follow up of surgically treated thyrotoxic patients. Br Med J 3:643, 1968.

19. Michie, W, Stowers, JM, Duncan, T, Pegg, CAS, et al.: Mechanism of hypocalcemia after thyroidectomy for thyrotoxicosis. Lancet 1:508, 1971.

20a. Blondeau, P, Brocard, M, Rene, L: Les Risques fonctionnels de la chirurgie thyroidienne. Ann Chir 27:1121, 1973.

20b. Bayley, TA, Harrison, JE, McNeill, KG, et al.: Effects of thyrotoxicosis and its treatment on bone mineral and muscle mass. J Clin Endocrinol Metab 50:916, 1980.

21. Miller, JM, Weber, RE, Block, MA: Treatment of hyperthyroidism from the autonomous multinodular goiter. Henry Ford Hosp. Med J 15:85, 1967.

22. Wilkin, TJ, Beck, JS, Michie, W: Does preoperative iodide treatment for thyrotoxicosis bring about involution? J Clin Pathol 30:99, 1977.

23. Cattell, RB: The pathology of exophthalmic goitre. Boston Medical and Surgical Journal 192:989, 1925.

24. Harden, R MCG, Koutras, DA, Alexander, WD, Wayne, EJ: Quantitative studies of iodine metabolism in iodine-treated thyrotoxicosis. Clin Sci 27:399, 1964.

25. Friend, DG: Iodide therapy and the importance of quantitating the dose. N Engl J Med 263:1358, 1960.

26. Bewsher, PD, Pegg, CA, Stewart, DJ, et al.: Propranolol in the surgical management of thyrotoxicosis. Ann Surg 180:787, 1974.

27. Caswell, HT, Marks, AD, Channick, BJ: Propranolol for the preoperative preparation of patients with thyrotoxicosis. Surg Gynecol Obstet 146:908, 1978.

28. Sawers, JSA, Toft, AD, Irvine, WJ, et al.: Transient hypothyroidism after Iodine-131 treatment of thyrotoxicosis, J Clin Endocrinol Metab 50:226, 1980.

APPENDIX: TECHNIQUE OF SURGERY

Saul Weinstein, M.D.

There are four types of surgical procedures today for the treatment of hyperthyroidism. The first, total lobectomy, is only suitable for the treatment of a toxic adenoma since it does not remove enough thyroid tissue to produce euthyroidism in Graves' disease. The other three procedures are suitable for the treatment of Graves' disease: 1) A subtotal thyroidectomy, leaving a rim of thyroid tissue on each side to protect the recurrent laryngeal nerves (bilateral, subtotal lobectomies and isthmusectomies) 2) Subtotal thyroidectomy, leaving only a small rim on one side (total thyroidectomy, isthmusectomy, and subtotal lobectomy on the opposite side), and 3) Total thyroidectomy.

Bilateral subtotal lobectomies, which usually leave 1/8-1/10 of the thyroid, do not require identification of the recurrent laryngeal nerve and thus for many surgeons the problem is "out of site and out of mind." Total lobectomy on one side, isthmusectomy, and subtotal lobectomy on the opposite side require identification of one recurrent laryngeal nerve but leave the oth other protected. This permits the surgeon to excise more thyroid tissue. The incidence of recurrence is less than with the bilateral subtotal lobectomies, but the incidence of permanent hypothyroidism and recurrent laryngeal nerve damage are greater. Total thyroidectomy uniformly produces hypothyroidism, but the patients are routinely started on thyroid replacement. In contrast after subtotal thyroidectomy the patients are not placed on thyroid replacement routinely and hypothyroidism often goes unrecognized. In addition after total thyroidectomy hyperthyroidism does not recur and thyroid ophthalmopathy does not usually progress. Only careful identification of both recurrent laryngeal nerves, both superior laryngeal nerves and the parathyroids will safely permit this procedure.

     As in most operations the following tenants of surgery are necessary. (1) good exposure (2) gentle handling of all tissues (3) thorough familiarization with the anatomy and identification of all vital structures prior to the removal of any tissue (4) proper lighting (5) adequate assistance and (6) good hemostasis. The operation is performed under general endotracheal anesthesia. The patient is in the supine position with the neck extended and a sand bag placed under the shoulders. The end of the table is elevated to prevent venous pooling in the operative area. To afford adequate exposure a transverse collar incision is made about 1-2 finger breadths above the sternoclavicular joint and extended from the anterior border of one sternocleidomastoid muscle to the same point on the opposite side. Placing the incision along a natural crease of the neck produces a satisfactory cosmetic result. The incision is then deepened through the platysma muscle. A majority of surgeons will develop skin flaps to enhance the exposure of the field. Thus the upper skin flap is raised to the level of the thyroid cartilage and the lower flap, to the sternoclavicular joints. On the other hand other surgeons will only raise the upper flap and some will develop none. Often times the troublesome bleeders in the undersurface of the flaps and in the skin margins will obscure the surgeon's view if not controlled. The dissection is now begun in the midline by dividing the fascia between the strap muscles. Here a decision must be made whether to retract or to divide these muscles. In dealing with toxic adenoma in which the size of the gland may be normal or slightly enlarged adequate exposure will be obtained by gentle retraction. When the gland is large or if bilateral nodularity exists then division of the strap muscles is necessary. There is little added morbidity when this is done in the postoperative period. The thyroid gland is now exposed and palpated. The next steps in the dissection will vary according to the requirements of the procedure and the preference of the surgeon. All have the following in common: (1) ligation of the middle thyroid veins, (2) identification of all four parathyroid glands and both recurrent laryngeal nerves, (3) identification of the descending branch of the superior laryngeal nerve, (4) ligation of the

Appendix: Technique of Surgery /69

superior thyroid vessels and (5) ligation of the inferior thyroid artery whenever the entire lob is to be removed.

The dissection continues by ligating the inferior thyroid suspensory ligament bearing the lower trachea to permit mobility of the lobe. Unless the pathology is confined to the left lobe it is the author's preference to begin the dissection on the right side. The middle thyroid vein is ligated to permit the surgeon to elevate and rotate the gland medially and to identify the recurrent laryngeal nerve and the inferior parathyroid gland. Attention is then directed to the upper pole where the superior thyroid vessels are located, doubly ligated and then divided as close as possible to the thyroid. This must follow identification of the descending branch of the superior laryngeal nerve.

The superior parathyroid gland and the terminal portion of the recurrent laryngeal nerve can be located by rotating and elevating the mobile right lobe medially. If the superior thyroid suspensory ligament has not been ligated it can be done at this point. All that remains is the separation of the lobe from its fibrous attachments to the trachea. As the gland is mobilized the dissection is continued from lateral to medial and from inferior to superior while keeping the parathyroids and recurrent laryngeal nerve in view always.

If the entire lobe is to be removed, the inferior thyroid artery is ligated prior to the freeing of the lobe from the trachea. As always the recurrent laryngeal nerve must be kept in view since it and the inferior thyroid artery may be closely related. To leave a small posterior portion of the lobe the thyroid artery is preserved and the dissection carried into the substance of the gland using straight hemostats to outline the line of resection.

As the medial portion of the lobe is freed from the trachea the isthmus is encountered. It is freed using electric cautery or clamp and tie techniques for hemostasis. The surgeon must be careful not to injure the trachea at this point. It is the author's preference to employ electric cautery liberally except in the area of the recurrent laryngeal nerve. There have been no complications following electric cautery and it facilitates rapid hemostasis with a minimum of effort to reduce operating time. If a pyramidal lobe is encountered it is removed in a similar fashion. Its point of origin in the area of the cricoid cartilage is usually ligated with a chromic suture.

With the right lobe, isthmus, and pyramidal lobe mobilized from the trachea attention is directed to the opposite lobe which is treated in a similar manner. The same careful dissection must be followed. The surgeon may leave a small posterior remnant of the left lobe by excising a portion of the gland or he may remove the entire lobe. The excised specimen is submitted to pathology for evaluation.

In anticipation of wound closure hemostasis is now checked. Once this has been accomplished drains are placed in the respective thyroid fossa and the strap muscles are approximated when necessary in the midline. The drains are brought out laterally between the strap muscle and the sternocleidomastoid to the surface. A suture or a safety pin will secure them to the most lateral portions of the skin incision. The platysma can be approximated with interrupted chromic sutures and the skin closed with either nonabsorbable sutures or metal clips. The application of a dressing completes the procedure.

When the patient is extubated an attempt may be made to examine the vocal cords, however, this is usually difficult and in some cases injury to the teeth occurs. Respiratory distress may develop immediately in the recovery room or over the course of the next several days. If it appears shortly after extubation then the following should be considered: (1) depressed respiratory reflexes from the effects of anesthesia (2) vocal paralysis from bilateral recurrent nerve paralysis or (3) edema of the vocal cords from trauma with the positioning of the endotracheal tube. A tracheostomy tray is kept at the bedside of the patient for the immediate postoperative period. When the respiratory distress is severe it is necessary to open the surgical incision to perform an immediate tracheostomy. Often it will not be possible to determine the etiology of the distress in these desperate situations. When secondary to the anesthesia a respiratory stimulant may also be required.

In less urgent situations indirect laryngoscopy may be helpful in assisting in the diagnosis of the source of the distress. Recurrent laryngeal paralysis or endotracheal tube trauma will produce vocal cords that remain in the midline and which are edematous with a minimal aperture. The airway can be established with an elective tracheostomy. Unilateral vocal cord paralysis usually causes impaired phonation. Dysfunction of the nerve may develop several days after surgery and probably represents neuropraxia from edema or stretching of the nerve. Repair will be necessary if evidence of damage persists for more than six months to a year following surgery.

Other causes of respiratory distress in the postoperative period include the following: (1) tracheal compression from hemorrhage or (2) tracheal collapse from instability of the cartilaginous rings. Hemorrhage should be expected when there is either swelling and discoloration of the wound and the patient is restless and has an increased pulse. It will be necessary to return the patient to surgery to control the bleeding and if necessary to insert a nasotracheal tube. Tracheal collapse may occur when a large gland causes weakening of the underlying tracheal rings. A tracheostomy must be performed above the softened area and a soft endotracheal tube passed to traverse this area. After several weeks the tube may be removed without the fear of future difficulties.

CHAPTER V

RADIOIODINE

At first glance radioiodine fits the concept of an ideal form of definitive therapy for the treatment of hyperthyroidism. Isotopes of iodine are accumulated and then incorporated into stored compounds only by the thyroid. Although several organs of the body as kidney, salivary glands, choroid plexus, and gastric mucosa trap iodine briefly, only the thyroid will receive substantial irradiation from a radioactive isotope of iodine. Treatment is convenient since suitable radioactive isotopes of iodine are easily administered orally. As a therapy radioiodine is far less expensive and more convenient than subtotal thyroidectomy. It does not require a prolonged course of administration as is necessary with the thioamides to achieve control of the hyperthyroidism. Unfortunately as clinical experience accumulated it became clear that while many of the complications of surgery and the thioamides were avoided radioiodine introduced a new set of complications. Thus these considerations narrow the selection of patients for radioiodine therapy of thyrotoxicosis.

This discussion will include the use of radioiodine as definitive therapy for hyperthyroidism as well as such complications as the production of hypothyroidism and the induction of thyroid carcinoma. In addition such problems as the effects on the bone marrow and gonads will also be covered. Such effects as a remission of the thyrotoxicosis appear first within a

matter of months. Within months to years hypothyroidism may
develop. After many years such potential problems as changes
produced in the bone marrow or the gonads may become apparent. Since the first reports of the use of radioiodine in the
early 1940's[1, 2] 131-iodine (^{131}I) has remained the isotope of
choice and this discussion will for the most part be limited to
its use.

MECHANISM OF ACTION

After a therapeutic dose of ^{131}I for the treatment of
hyperthyroidism, there may be no histologic changes discernable in the thyroid even though euthyroidism has been achieved.[3]
In some the changes will consist only of involution of the hyperplastic cells. With doses of ^{131}I far larger than those used in
the treatment of thyrotoxicosis changes as obvious epithelial
injury and a necrotic vasculitis are seen. Follicular injury and
perifollicular fibrosis follow. Hence the effect of radioiodine
in hyperthyroidism must be more complex than just a uniform
destruction of thyroid cells. The success of ^{131}I ablation undoubtedly stems from the irregular accumulation of iodine by
the thyroid. Any one of a number of investigators have demonstrated that iodine is distributed in a heterologous fashion reflecting differences in follicular iodine concentration as well as
variation in the distribution of the follicles throughout the
thyroid.[4] Hence for any dose of radioiodine there will be marked
variation in the radiation exposure from follicle to follicle.
Some follicles will receive a radiation dose that may exceed the
dose calculated for the thyroid as a whole while other follicles
may receive hardly any irradiation. The net effect is thus a
selective thyroid ablation.

The appearance of hypothyroidism months to years
after the administration of a therapeutic dose of ^{131}I may be a
consequence of sublethal damage to the nucleus.[5] Enough
thyroid cells survive the radiation damage to maintain euthyroidism. Yet these cells either survive for a shorter period
than usual or fail to divide. Eventually the number of cells will
be inadequate to maintain normal thyroid function.

Iodine-125 (^{125}I) was used in the therapy of hyperthyroidism to avoid the production of hypothyroidism. This isotope has a half-life of 60. 2 days and is considered a pure emitter of gamma rays. In the transformation to its more stable
isotope electrons are produced that travel only from within the
colloid to the colloid-follicular cell interface,[6] the site of

hormonal production. The isotope ^{131}I emits gamma rays which pass relatively unabsorbed through the thyroid and beta particles which travel a maximum distance of 2 mm within the thyroid.[7] The radiation of ^{125}I should be delivered primarily to that portion of the follicle most active in the synthesis of thyroid hormones (colloid-cell interface) whereas ^{131}I will deliver radiation to a far wider area (colloid and cell). Unfortunately the incidence of hypothyroidism is not lower after ^{125}I ablation so that though the proportion of irradiation delivered to the nucleus is small, it is still sufficient to produce hypothyroidism.[8] What is more hypothyroidism may actually occur more frequently after the use of ^{125}I than with ^{131}I. Hypothyroidism is thus an inescapable consequence of radioiodine therapy irrespective of the isotope employed.

SELECTION OF PATIENTS

Radioiodine is absolutely contraindicated in pregnancy and relatively contraindicated in children. Once the fetal thyroid begins to accumulate iodine after the twelfth week of gestation[9] there is the problem of damage to the fetal thyroid. Iodine crosses the placenta regardless of the isotope and thus the radioactive isotopes will deliver a substantial dose of irradiation to the fetal thyroid. With the size of the dose in the treatment of thyrotoxicosis there is little question that ablation of the fetal thyroid will occur as well. Furthermore the use of any form of radiation in pregnancy always brings up the possibility of inducing some cellular damage in the fetus that may not appear until many years later. Whenever any doubt exists about the possibility of pregnancy it is imperative to obtain a pregnancy test before administering a dose of ^{131}I either for the purpose of diagnostic studies or for ablating the thyroid. Should the accident occur most physicians allow the pregnancy to continue to term.[10] Although the incidence of abortions and congenital anomalies differ little from normal pregnancies, there is little information about the long term effects on these offspring. Hypothyroidism and mental retardation occurred far more frequently in these children than might have been expected following uncomplicated pregnancies. It is imperative that such children be observed most carefully for hypothyroidism.

The following case illustrates the problem of the administration of ^{131}I to a patient whose pregnancy was unsuspected. The diagnosis of hyperthyroidism was established in this 33-year-old patient in August, 1976. She had undergone a tubal ligation following her last pregnancy seven years previously. Symptoms, present for about one month, included pruritis, weight loss, and extreme irritability. Ablation with ^{131}I was elected as the means of definitive therapy and the patient received 6 mCi in August. Within two weeks of the administration of the radioiodine it became apparent that the patient was pregnant. Careful review of her history elicited the fact that her menses which were ordinarily quite regular had ceased in June, 1976.

The problems of continuing the pregnancy were carefully reviewed for the patient and she decided to continue the pregnancy. Between August and the birth of the child in March by Cesarian section she remained free of the symptoms of hyperthyroidism. It was not necessary to use any medication to control symptoms and her T4 remained in the normal range for pregnancy. The patient has remained euthyroid so far; however, the child was found to be hypothyroid at one month of age.

The case illustrates that a careful menstrual history is imperative whenever a radioactive isotope is to be used in a woman during her reproductive years. In this case the tubal ligation provided a false sense of security and test for pregnancy was certainly warranted. At the very least another form of therapy for the hyperthyroidism should have been selected. Control of the hyperthyroidism could not have been achieved any more easily with either surgery or a thioamide. The dose of radioiodine, average by any means of calculation, was administered at the very time which the fetal thyroid begins to accumulate iodine. Subsequent observation confirmed the fear of fetal thyroid ablation. Hopefully the benefits gained in the treatment of the mother will not be achieved at the cost of problems for the child.

Arguments for the use of radioiodine in children can be quite persuasive.[10] The incidence of permanent remission compares favorably with surgery or a course of a thioamide. Over a long period of follow up the fertility rate of these patients and the incidence of spontaneous abortion in pregnancies of these patients does not differ from normal. Thyroid nodules do appear following the use of ^{131}I in children for the treatment of hyperthyroidism. However, nearly all of these nodules were benign when examined following a subtotal thyroidectomy.[12] Unfortunately this fear of thyroid malignancy still lingers in spite of this evidence. This plus the substantial risk of hypothyroidism and the need for life-long thyroid replacement following therapy with ^{131}I in a substantial proportion of children make it less attractive for treating the hyperthyroid child. The child with a severe concurrent medical problem will still be a candidate for radioiodine.

The physical characteristics of the goiter have been used in the selection of a form of definitive therapy to influence the choice of ^{131}I as the modality. When the thyroid is sufficiently large to produce symptoms of compression, a relatively rare problem in hyperthyroidism, the treatment should be surgery. Neither the rate at which thyroid size decreases nor the total reduction in thyroid size are certain enough with ^{131}I to use it in these circumstances. Another indication for surgery is thyroid nodularity. It has been argued that since these patients are often poor medical risks and since large doses of ^{131}I are required, often over an extended period, surgery is preferable by producing euthyroidism most rapidly.[13] Yet a thioamide can be used to quickly render such patients euthyroid so that ^{131}I can be administered when the hyperthyroidism is controlled. Additional doses of radioiodine can be repeated while control is maintained with the thioamide, and the symptoms of hyperthyroidism should not be a problem regardless of the time required for ^{131}I to produce its effect. Experience with ^{131}I in this situation has been quite favorable.[14] Furthermore the concept of thyroid nodularity is far more complex than once thought.[15] On careful scrutiny of nodular goiters there is a spectrum from diffuse involvement of all follicles to the involvement of multiple individual follicles. The question then is whether one type of nodularity warrants special therapeutic consideration. For the most part the physical characteristics of the thyroid will rarely dictate the modality of therapy to the exclusion of other features.

The ideal candidates for ^{131}I include the following: (1) patients over 40, (2) adults with complicating illness as lesions of the cardiac valves, or a problem as Sickle Cell Disease, (3) adults with a recurrence following surgery, and (4) patients with a sensitivity to the available thioamides. It is not easy to prove that age 40 is better than age 30 in selecting radioiodine as definitive therapy. This choice will depend on such considerations as the problems of neoplasia and the fears of gonadal damage. Some guidelines will be discussed in the section on complications. The ease of the administration of ^{131}I provides a convenient means of treating thyrotoxicosis, for example, in the presence of congestive heart failure. The therapeutic dose may be given during the therapy of the heart failure or the patient can be treated briefly with a thioamide beforehand to produce symptomatic relief. When the hyperthyroidism recurs following subtotal thyroidectomy it is customary to treat the patient with ^{131}I. Usually these patients have chosen surgery to avoid a course of a thioamide so that with recurrence this modality is not appropriate. Surgery is not an attractive alternative either since most patients who undergo a second thyroidectomy will usually recur.[16] Until the availability of propranolol sensitivity to a thioamide usually precluded surgery in the past as there was no alternative, safe way to prepare such patients for surgery. Radioiodine, however, for most patients sensitive to thioamides, still will be the best alternative. Table V.1 lists the exclusions and indications for the use of radioiodine.

TABLE V.1

INDICATIONS AND EXCLUSION FOR
ABLATION WITH ^{131}I IN HYPERTHYROIDISM

EXCLUDE	ABSOLUTE	Pregnant patients
	RELATIVE	Children
INCLUDE WITH RESERVATIONS		Adolescents with a concurrent illness (i.e., Sickle Cell Disease)
		Multinodular goiter
		Uncooperative patient
INCLUDE AS IDEAL		Patients over 40 Adults with complicating illness as congestive heart failure. With recurrence following surgery. When sensitivity to a thioamide.

The following case illustrates the use of ^{131}I and propylthiouracil in a 54-year-old woman with severe hyperthyroidism. Beginning in January, 1978, the patient complained of increased weakness, recurrent ankle edema, increased sweating, heat intolerance, weight loss, and dyspnea climbing stairs. When first seen in May, 1978, the physical findings included a thyroid three times normal in size, a summation gallop, inability to arise from a chair, and massive pretibial edema. The T4 was 22 mcg% (Normal 5-12), a T3-resin 60% (Normal 25-35%), and the 24-hour thyroid uptake 70% (Normal 10-35%). Because of her very precarious state the patient was admitted to the hospital for therapy. Her condition stabilized sufficiently over the first 5 days following admission with the use of digitalis and furosemide so that it was possible to administer 7 miC ^{131}I. Three days later propylthiouracil was started using 100 mg three times daily. Over the next two months the patients' symptoms slowly subsided and her weight increased by 10 pounds. Three months after the dose of ^{131}I a T4 was 5.9 mcg%. In September, 1978 the propylthiouracil was stopped for three days and the thyroid uptake repeated. It was 56% and a second therapeutic dose of ^{131}I was administered. Three days later the propylthiouracil was restarted.

The severity of the thyrotoxicosis had progressed in this patient so that it was necessary to admit her for the control of the cardiac symptoms. The patient had improved so remarkably that it was possible to administer radioiodine ablation before beginning a thioamide. Ordinarily one would place the patient on the thioamide for several weeks to allow depletion of thyroid hormone stores. The interval of 3 days between the dose of ^{131}I and the start of PTU allowed sufficient recirculation of the isotope before blocking further iodine uptake. The addition of PTU this rapidly allowed the patient to become euthyroid as quickly as possible and to remain euthyroid regardless of the success of the first dose of radioiodine in controlling the hyperthyroidism. In such precarious patients there seems little reason to allow the symptoms of hyperthyroidism to recur, or for that matter, to demand that the T4 be elevated before considering retreatment with ^{131}I. An elevated thyroid uptake is sufficient for the diagnosis. As a matter of policy there seems little reason to allow severe symptoms to persist in most patients and control should be attempted with either a thioamide or propranolol.

SELECTION OF A DOSE OF ^{131}I

Once it has been decided to treat the hyperthyroidism with ^{131}I, there may be a question of the timing of the first dose as in the patient with severe cardiovascular disease. For the usual hyperthyroid patient the dose of radioiodine can be administered as soon as the diagnosis is established.[17] When there is concern about the safety of ^{131}I with regard to the production of a radiation thyroiditis and the release of stored hormones, the following procedure should suffice: following the diagnosis of hyperthyroidism, PTU is started at 100 mg every 8 hours and continued for 6 weeks. Then the patient is taken off the thioamide, the thyroid uptake performed and the dose of ^{131}I administered. The PTU is then restarted after 3-5 days and the cycle repeated until the thyroid uptake returns to normal.

The use of a thioamide either before the dose of ^{131}I or afterward permits more rapid depletion of the stores of the thyroid hormones. Symptoms are controlled far more quickly than with radioiodine alone. A thioamide will usually control the hyperthyroidism within 6 weeks whereas ^{131}I often requires 3 months. One objection to the combined use of a thioamide and ^{131}I is that thioamides may exert a protective effect against the radiation.[18] This might be significant if more or larger doses of ^{131}I are required, if the course after radioiodine is altered, if remission is delayed, or if the incidence of hypothyroidism is altered. There has been little difference in the outcome when a thioamide has been employed along with ^{131}I and this fear is unsupported by actual clinical experience.[14]

It usually requires 6 weeks to 3 months for the full effect of a dose of ^{131}I to appear. Many will wait as long as 6 months in hopes of avoiding the occurrence of hypothyroidism. It is the author's preference to plan to retreat the patient at the 3 month interval. If the patient can be controlled on propranolol then the usual parameters of thyroid function will indicate whether or not a remission has occurred. Persistance of symptoms will also indicate this. When a thioamide has been used to block the symptoms it is only necessary to withhold the medication for 3-5 days before repeating the thyroid uptake. An elevated uptake can be used as an indication for retreating the patient. This course can be repeated until euthyroidism is achieved. If one chooses to wait 6 months then the patient's symptoms can be blocked with propranolol or a thioamide. It has been the author's experience that this tends to prolong treatment far too long and really will not alter the incidence of hypothyroidism.

There have been many formulas used to calculate the dose of ^{131}I since this therapy was first introduced. Most formulas reflect an empirical derivation for the delivery of a dose of radiation. Furthermore these are based on assumptions made about the actual distribution of the radioactive isotope, and the rate at which iodine actually enters and leaves the gland. Needless to say estimation of thyroid size is only an approximation. The most satisfactory solution, one that accepts many of these limitations, attempts to deliver 80-160μCi ^{131}I/gram of thyroid (retained). This dose of radiation has achieved the most satisfactory results as any one of a number of surveys demonstrate.[19] The range allows some flexibility so that a smaller dose is available for the average patient and a larger dose for the patient in whom control is desirable with the least number of doses. Sixty percent of all patients require only a single dose of ^{131}I and ninety per cent will undergo a remission with the second dose.

Table V.2 illustrates the differences in the dose of radiation delivered to the thyroid using three levels of doses of ^{131}I. The calculations are based on a thyroid of 40 grams with an uptake of 60% at 24 hours. The range varies from the low of 50μCi ^{131}I delivered to 200μCi. It should be evident from this table that higher doses of ^{131}I improve the rate of remission but also increase the incidence of hypothyroidism. Furthermore this improvement in the rate of hypothyroidism is followed by an unacceptable rate of remission at these lower doses. In other words the case for a dose of radioiodine below 80μCi per gram is not very convincing. At the range of $80-160\mu$Ci ^{131}I there is little evidence that delaying retreatment beyond 3 months and using a thioamide or propranolol influences the incidence of hypothyroidism.

TABLE V.2

A COMPARISON OF VARIOUS DOSES OF ^{131}I ON THE INCIDENCE OF HYPOTHYROIDISM AND HYPERTHYROIDISM

Dose	μCi ^{131}I/g thyroid (Retained)	Total Dose	Patients Remaining Hyperthyroid at one year (%)	Patients Hypothyroid at one year (%)
Low	50	3.3	54.1%	7.1%
Standard	80	5.3	23	6
High	160-200	13.3	10	26

These calculations are derived from references 20, 21, and 22 and are based on a 40 gram thyroid with an uptake of 60% at 24 hours.

A prepresentative case using ^{131}I therapy is as follows: The patient, a 70-year-old male was first evaluated in July, 1977 because of weight loss, increased nervousness, increased sweating, and diarrhea. The thyroid was twice normal in size, the pulse, 100/minute. A T4 was 12.5 mcg% (normal 5-12), a T3 resin uptake 38% (normal 25-35%), a T3 by radioimmunoassay 260 ng% (normal 60-190). Thyroid uptake at 24 hours was 38%. The patient was given 6 μCi ^{131}I in August. His symptoms disappeared over the next 3 months so that by November he was free of complaints. His weight had increased by 8 pounds. A T4 was 8 mcg% and the T3 by radioimmunoassay 160 ng%. Since then he has remained euthyroid.

The case illustrates the appearance of hyperthyroidism as T3-thyrotoxicosis. The symptoms were sufficiently mild so that it was not necessary to use either propranolol or a thioamide for control of symptoms. The course to euthyroidism was smooth following a conventional dose of 80 μCi ^{131}I (retained). The appearance of hypothyroidism will always be a consideration during the lifetime of the patient.

COMPLICATIONS

Exacerbation of hyperthyroidism and thyroid storm[23] represent rare potential problems following ^{131}I therapy. Thyroid storm has been reported so infrequently that its occurrence can be considered unimportant. The exacerbation of hyperthyroidism has been attributed to the release of stored hormones with radiation damage. As noted earlier there is often no evidence of microscopic changes with ^{131}I and only much larger doses damaging the follicles sufficiently to cause release of colloid. Surprisingly most patients tolerate the symptoms of hyperthyroidism well so that unless there is a concurrent problem as congestive failure this exacerbation should not be of great concern.

Hypothyroidism is an inevitable complication of ^{131}I therapy. Reducing the dose of ^{131}I only delays its appearance. The early appearance of hypothyroidism with a dose as low as 50 μCi is lower than with doses above this range but the cumulative incidence still remains similar.[24,25,26] About 7-10% of patients become hypothyroid in the first year after a dose of 80-160 μCi and the yearly incidence thereafter is 2-3%. A curve which plots the appearance of hypothyroidism against the year of follow up continues upward for as long as patients are followed.[27,28] In theory at least all will eventually become hypothyroid. It has been suggested recently that the incidence of hypothyroidism may actually be as high as 70% after one year.[29] The cumulative incidence of hypothyroidism for the most part remains independent of the number of treatments. After four or more doses of ^{131}I the occurrence of hypothyroidism is less frequent than with fewer doses. The incidence of hypothyroidism with ^{125}I may actually be higher than with ^{131}I.[30]

It would be useful if there were a means of identifying when patients will become hypothyroid. There is no substitute for careful followup after ^{131}I therapy. The patient would understand that the followup must continue indefinitely. The clinical impression can be confirmed by a low T4. Levels of thyrotropin (TSH) may be elevated after ^{131}I therapy, but all such patients are not hypothyroid.[31] Values of triiodothyronine (T3) determined by radioimmunoassay do not always correlate with the clinical state.[32] Many patients are hypothyroid yet T3 falls into the normal range. In the euthyroid patients the response of TSH to thyrotropin releasing factor has also not helped in predicting the onset of hypothyroidism.[33] Patients are more apt to develop hypothyroidism if cytoplasmic antibodies appear after radioiodine therapy,[34] but diagnosis must still be based on clinical evidence. Addition of thyroid supplement as soon as euthyroidism is achieved avoids the appearance of hypothyroidism. However, this can complicate the followup since if symptoms of hyperthyroidism appear it is not always clear whether the hyperthyroidism has recurred or if the dose of thyroid replacement is excessive.

In deciding about radioiodine there has been some concern that the ophthalmopathy of Graves' disease will deteriorate following treatment.[35] Chapter VII covers this problem in detail. There is little evidence that progression of these manifestations occur in response to ^{131}I therapy. It is usually far more important to render the patient euthyroid since most therapies directed at the eye complications require that the patient be euthyroid.

The following case illustrates the importance of careful follow up after radioiodine ablation. The patient, a 75-year-old woman, complained of poor energy, impaired memory, cold intolerance, dry skin, and severe constipation. She had received a dose of ^{131}I for hyperthyroidism nearly twenty years previously. In the interval the patient had been hospitalized many times for severe depression. The thyroid was twice normal in size, pulse 60/minute; skin was coarse, cool, and dry. Her reflexes were myotonic. A T4 was 1.5 mcg% (normal 5-12) and a TSH 30 μu/ml (normal less than 10). The patient was started on thyroid replacement and her depression improved. However the appearance of angina prevented full replacement so that euthyroidism was not achieved.

Unfortunately the patient was not informed of the need for continued follow up. Hypothyroidism appeared and remained undetected through most of her psychiatric illness. That most of her depression could have been avoided with prompt replacement of thyroid hormone remains moot but certainly worthy of discussion. As in so many of these patients full replacement was not tolerated.

Since ^{131}I circulates through the body before its incorporation into hormone by the thyroid and its excretion by the kidney, its use raises the question of the induction of neoplasia in organs other than the thyroid. The importance of the observations of chromosomal abnormalities following ^{131}I is not clear but does suggest that there may be some effect on nonthyroid cells. Figure 5.1 depicts in a diagramatic fashion the problem of radiation exposure from ^{131}I to the various organs of the body. Since much of the data has been derived from euthyroid models the results can be viewed only in a relative fashion rather than as absolute values for the number of rads delivered in the treatment of hypothyroidism. As a consequence of such exposure problems as thyroid carcinoma, parathyroid damage, laryngeal carcinoma, genetic damage and leukemia must be considered. There is in addition the problem of the radiation hazard to other individuals.

It has been recognized for sometime that thyroid nodules appear after ^{131}I therapy in the child and the adolescent patient.[40] When removed most of these nodules were benign; however, a few were thyroid carcinomas. In a group of 256 patients thyroid nodules appeared in 8 patients, and two were thyroid carcinoma. No nodules were found in patients over 30 years of age. The most recent experience[11] with the use of ^{131}I in the treatment of hyperthyroidism in childhood has not encountered the problem of thyroid nodules with long term follow up. A recent cooperative study[41] investigated the problem of malignant and benign neoplasms following the use of ^{131}I. There were 86 malignant neoplasms in a group of 34,684 patients treated by several modalities. The incidence of malignant neoplasms in the patients treated by ^{131}I did not differ from that in patients treated with subtotal thyroidectomy.

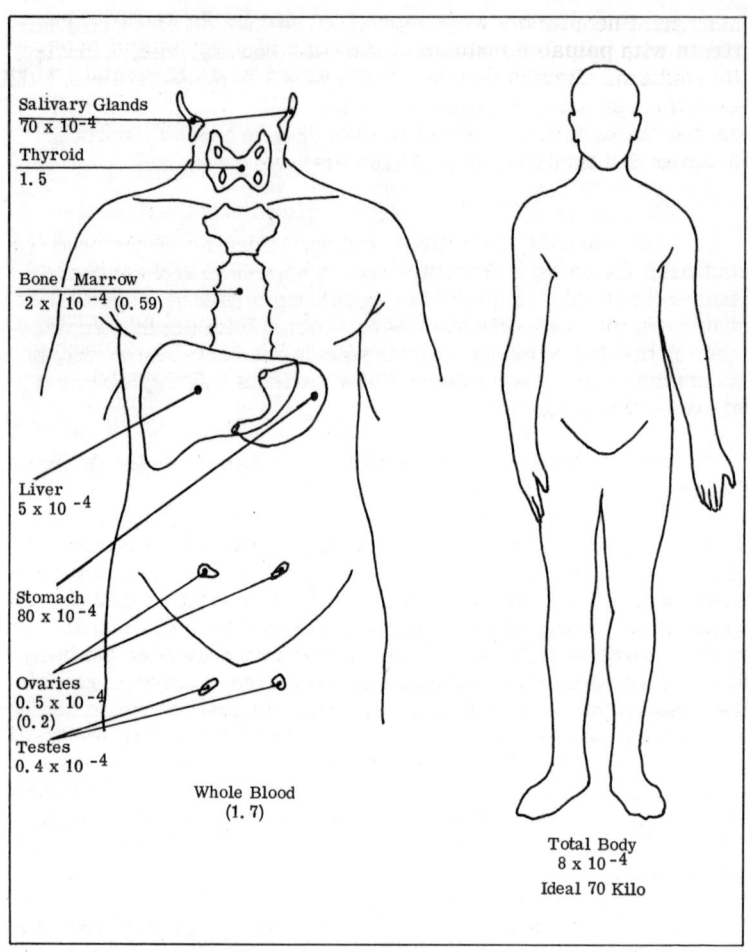

FIGURE 5.1: Radiation Exposure From ^{131}I to Various Body Organs

ORGAN

RADS/μCl ^{131}I administered

The figure is derived from data provided in references 36-39. The figures, except when noted in parenthesis, have been derived from euthyroid models and are thus only relative expressions of radiation exposure in hyperthyroid patients.

Malignant neoplasms were more frequent in the group of patients with palpable nodules at the time of diagnosis of hyperthyroidism. Benign neoplasms occurred more frequently when ^{131}I therapy was administered to patients in the first two decades of life. Thus for the adult the risk of thyroid carcinoma after ^{131}I therapy for hyperthyroidism is negligible.

The use of ^{131}I also raises the question of the induction of neoplasia in organs other than the thyroid. Chromosomal abnormalities do occur following ^{131}I.[42] Although there have been case reports of leukemia following ^{131}I, there is no evidence that leukemia is any more frequent after radioiodine therapy than it is after subtotal thyroidectomy.[44] Surprisingly the occurrence is far more common after both of these modalities of therapy than in a control population. The dose of radiation to the bone marrow with ^{131}I has been calculated at 0.59 rads/μCi ^{131}I administered.[37] This dose is probably not significant with regard to the problem of bone marrow changes.

One of the reasons for excluding patients in the reproductive years is the fear of producing genetic damage through irradiation to the gonads. It has been estimated that a 10 mCi dose of ^{131}I delivers 3.2 rads to the gonads.[39] By comparison such radiological procedures as a barium enema, an intravenous urogram, or a hysterosalpingography deliver at least this amount of irradiation, and in some cases even more. The risks have undoubtedly been overstated in light of all of the evidence accumulated so far. Neither theoretical considerations nor clinical observations support this fear. If children are followed after receiving ^{131}I into reproductive life, there is no evidence that there has been any such damage.[12] It cannot be denied however that this fear makes radioiodine an unattractive choice for therapy regardless of such evidence in the younger patient.

SUMMARY

Figure 5.2 outlines the use of radioiodine in the form of a flow diagram. It is the author's view that ^{131}I therapy in hyperthyroidism does not induce carcinoma of the thyroid, nor induce leukemia or genetic damage. It is the author's habit to use ^{131}I as the first choice of definitive therapy in patients over forty, in younger patients when other modalities are unsuitable, in patients with a recurrence of thyrotoxicosis following subtotal

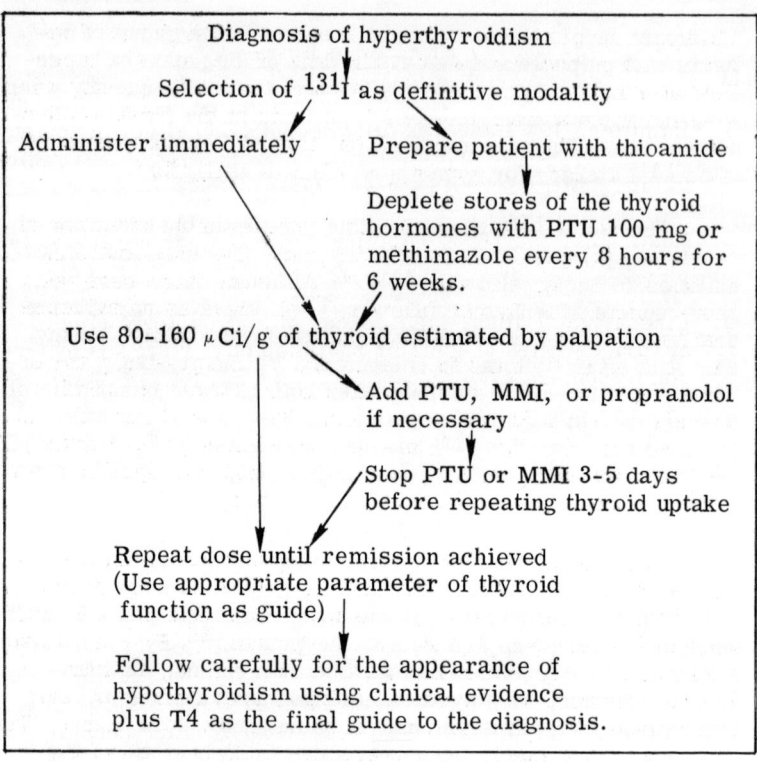

FIGURE 5.2: Outlining of the use of ^{131}I in treating hyperthyroidism

thyroidectomy, and in the patients who have a serious complicating illness at any age. With rare exceptions either a thioamide or propranolol are used to control the symptoms of hyperthyroidism until a remission of the hyperthyroidism occurs. The initial dose of ^{131}I must be sufficiently large to produce the highest rate of remission as well as the smallest possible initial rate of hypothyroidism. With this aim in mind the occurrence of hypothyroidism in a proportion of the patients is inevitable. It is essential that follow up be continued indefinitely.

REFERENCES

1. Hamilton, JC, Larence, JH: Recent clinical developments in the therapeutic application of radiophosphorus and radioiodine. J Clin Invest 21:624, 1942.

2. Hertz, S, Roberts, S: Application of radioactive iodine in therapy of Graves' disease. J Clin Invest 21:624, 1942.

3. Lindsay, S, Dailey, ME, Jones, MD: Histologic effects of various types of ionizing radiation on normal and hyperplastic human thyroid glands. J Clin Endocrinol Metab 14:1179, 1954.

4. Clayton, CG: Irregularities of iodine assimulation by the follicles of the rat thyroid. Br J Radiol 26:99, 1953.

5. Grieg, WR: Radiation, thyroid cells and ^{131}I therapy A hypothysis. J Clin Endocrinol Metab 25:1411, 1965.

6. Lewitus, Z, Lubin, E, Rechnic, J, Ben-Porath, M, Feige, Y: Treatment of thyrotoxicosis with ^{125}I and ^{131}I. Semin Nucl Med 1:411, 1971.

7. Dillman, LT: Radionuclide decay schemes and nuclear parameters for use in radiation-dose estimation. J Nucl Med 10:Supplement No. 2, 1969 (NM/MIRD pamphlet, No. 4)

8. Bremner, WF, McDougall, IR, Greig, WR: Results of treating 297 thyrotoxic patients with ^{125}I. Lancet 2:281, 1973.

9. Chapman, EM, Corner, GW Jr, Robinson, D, Evans, RD: The collection of radioactive iodine by the human fetal thyroid. J Clin Endocrinol Metab 8:717, 1948.

10. Stoffer, SS, Hamburger, JI: Inadvertent ^{131}I therapy for hyperthyroidism in the first trimester of pregnancy. J Nucl Med 17:146, 1976.

11. Safa, AM, Schumacher, OP, Rodriguez-Antunez, A: Long-term follow-up results in children and adolescents treated with radioactive iodine (^{131}I) for hyperthyroidism. N Engl J Med 292:167, 1975.

12. Starr, R, Jaff, HL, Oettinger, L: Later results of ^{131}I treatment of hyperthyroidism in 73 children and adolescents:1967 follow-up. J Nucl Med 10:586, 1969.

13. Miller, JM: Radioiodine therapy of the autonomous functioning thyroid. Semin Nucl Med 1:43, 1971.

14. Lomberg, BA, Hernberg, CA, Wahlberg, P, et al.: Treatment of toxic nodular goiter with radioiodine. Acta Med Scan 165:245, 1959.

15. Studer, H, Hunziker, HR, Ruchti, C: Morphologic and functional substrate of thyrotoxicosis caused by nodular goiters. Am J Med 65:227, 1978.

16. Kalk, WJ, Kantor, S, Durbach, D, et al.: Post-thyroidectomy thyrotoxicosis. Lancet 1:291, 1978.

17. Becker, DV, Hurley, Jr: Complications of radioiodine treatment of hyperthyroidism. Sem Nucl Med 1:442, 1971.

18. Goolden, AWG, Fraser, TR: Effect of pretreatment with carbimazole in patients with thyrotoxicosis subsequently treated with radioactive iodine. Br M J 3:442, 1969.

19. Beierwaltes, WH: The treatment of hyperthyroidism with iodine-181. Semin Nucl Med 8:95, 1978.

20. Hagen, GA, Ouellette, RP, Chapman, EM: Comparison of high and low dosage levels of ^{131}I in the treatment of thyrotoxicosis. N Engl J Med 277:559, 1967.

21. Rapoport, B, Caplan, RL, DeGroot, LJ: Low dose sodium iodine ^{131}I therapy in Graves' disease. JAMA 224:1610, 1973.

22. Safa, AM, Skillern, PG: Treatment of hyperthyroidism with a large initial dose of sodium 131. Arch Int Med 135:673, 1975.

23. Shafter, RB, Nuttall, RQ: Acute changes in thyroid function in patients treated with radioactive iodine. Lancet 2:635, 1975.

24. Cervallos, JL, Hagen, GA, Maloot, F, Chapman, EM: Low dose 131 therapy of thyrotoxicosis. N Engl J Med 290:191, 1974.

25. Rappaport, B, Caplan, R, DeGroot, LJ: Low dose sodium iodine I 131 therapy in Graves' disease. JAMA 224:1610, 1973.

26. Nofa, M, Beierwates, WH, Patno, ME: Treatment of hyperthyroidism with sodium iodine I-131. JAMA 197:87, 1966.

27. Dunn, JT, Chapman, EM: Rising incidence of hyperthyroidism after radioactive-iodine therapy in thyrotoxicosis. N Engl J Med 271:1037, 1964.

28. Einhorn, J, Wicklund, H: Hypothyroidism following ^{131}I treatment for hyperthyroidism. J Clin Endocrinol Metab 26:33, 1966.

29. Vanhofe, SE, Dorfman, SG, Carretta, RF, Young, RL: The increasing incidence of hypothyroidism within one year after radioiodine therapy for toxic diffuse goiter. J Nucl Med 19:180, 1978.

30. McDougall, IR, Greig, WR: ^{125}I therapy in Graves' disease. Long-term results in 355 patients. Ann Intern Med 85:720, 1976.

31. Toft, AD, Hunter, WM, Seth, J, Irvine, WJ: Plasma-thyrotropin and serum-thyroxine in patients becoming hypothyroid in the early months after iodine-131. Lancet 1: 704, 1974.

32. Tunbridge, WMG, Harsoulis, P, Goolden, AWG: Thyroid function in patients treated with radioactive iodine for thyrotoxicosis. Br Med J 3:89, 1974.

33. Gordin, A, Wagar, G, Henberg, A: Serum thyrotropin and response to thyrotropin-releasing hormone in patients who are euthyroid after radioiodine treatment for hyperthyroidism. Acta Med Scand 194:335, 1973.

34. Lundell, G, Jonsson, J: Thyroid antibodies and hypothyroidism in ^{131}I therapy for hyperthyroidism. Acta Radiol 12:443, 1973.

35. Weidinger, P, Johnson, PM, Werner, SC: Five years' experience with iodine - 125 therapy of Graves' disease. Lancet 2:74, 1974.

36. Willman, HN, Anger, RJ, Jr: Radioiodine Dosimetry and the use of radioiodine other than ^{131}I in thyroid diagnosis. Sem Nucl Med 1:3566, 1971.

37. McEwan, AC: Absorbed doses in the marrow during ^{131}I therapy. Br J Radio 50:329, 1977.

38. Green, M, Fisher, M, Miller, H, Wilson, GM: Blood radiation dose after ^{131}I therapy of thyrotoxicosis. Br Med J 2:210, 1961.

39. Robertson, JS, Gorman, CA: Gonadal radiation dose and its genetic significance in radioiodine therapy of hyperthyroidism. J Nucl Med 17:826, 1976.

40. Sheline, GE, Lindsay, S, McCormack, KR, Galante, M: Thyroid nodules occurring late after treatment of thyrotoxicosis with radioiodine. J Clin Endocrinol Metab 22: 8, 1962.

41. Dobyns, BM, Sheline, GE, Workman, JB, Tompkins, EA, McConahey, WM, Becker, DV: Malignant and benign neoplasms of the thyroid in patients treated for hyperthyroidism: A report of the cooperative thyrotoxicosis therapy follow-up study. J Clin Endocrinol Metab 38:976, 1974.

42. Cantolino, SJ, Schmickel, RD, Ball, M, Cisar, CF: Persistent chromosomal aberrations following radioiodine therapy for thyrotoxicosis, N Engl J Med 275:739, 1966.

43. Pochin, EE, Myant, NB, Corbett, BD: Leukemia following radioiodine treatment of hyperthyroidism. Br J Radiol 29: 3135, 1956.

44. Saenger, EL, Thoma, GE, Tompkins, EA: Incidence of leukemia following treatment of hyperthyroidism. JAMA 205:855, 1968.

CHAPTER VI

HYPERTHYROIDISM IN CHILDHOOD

Thomas Moshang, M. D.

During childhood, hyperfunctioning of the thyroid gland is usually due to Graves' Disease, although thyroiditic (Hashimoto's) thyrotoxicosis is occasionally encountered. Hyperfunctioning nodules are much less common and hyperthyroidism secondary to overproduction of thyrotropin (TSH) is extremely rare. Therefore, this discussion of therapeutic modalities will be directed towards the hyperthyroid newborn infant and the child with classic Graves' Disease.

NEONATAL HYPERTHYROIDISM

The hyperthyroid neonate will invariably be the infant of a mother with either active Graves' Disease or a past history of Graves' Disease. All of these infants will have enlargement of their thyroid glands, large soft goiters. However, because the mothers will often have been on antithyroid medication, it is difficult to ascertain whether the goiter is secondary to antithyroid medication or thyrostimulating immunoglobulins (or some other factor). Both cross the placental barrier. Parenthetically, thyroxine (T4) and triiodothyronine (T3) do not appear to pass from the mother to the fetus. The difficulties in establishing the diagnosis of neonatal hyperthyroidism is compounded by the fact that all normal term newborns are biochemically thyrotoxic (Table VI. 1)[1, 2, 3]

TABLE VI. 1

THYROID HORMONE LEVELS IN TERM NEWBORNS[1, 2, 3]

Age	T_4 (ugm/dl) mean	T_4 (ugm/dl) range	T_3 (ngm/dl) mean	TSH (uU/dl) mean
Cord	10.9	7.3 - 15.3	48	8.5
2 hrs.	22.1		217	
3 days	17.2	10.1 - 21.4	125	7.3
6 wks.	10.3	7.5 - 16.6	163	2.5

T_4 levels increase rapidly in newborn children, peaking to levels greater than 20 ugm/dl in the first several hours and then slowly declining over the next several months. Inasmuch as T_4 levels in thyrotoxic newborns are often within the upper limits of the normal range of values, T_4 determinations may not establish the diagnosis of neonatal hyperthyroidism. However, since the infant with a goiter secondary to maternal ingestion of antithyroid medication would be expected to have low normal values of T_4, high T_4 values do help confirm clinical findings of hyperthyroidism. T_3 values normally decline more rapidly (the mean T_3 level for 3-day-old children is 125 ngm/dl but a number of normal 3-day-old newborn infants will continue to have T_3 levels greater than 200 ngm/dl. Furthermore, the time interval required for the return of the results of special thyroid function tests, such as T_3, TSH or free T_4, make these tests less useful in the clinical situation of a thyrotoxic newborn.

All infants born to a mother actively hyperthyroid or with a past history of Graves' disease is at risk for neontal thyrotoxicosis. The diagnosis of neonatal thyrotoxicosis is based on the clinical manifestations and supported by the laboratory finding of high normal or elevated T_4 values. The clinical manifestations include poor weight gain or weight loss, tachycardia, flushing, irritability, jitteriness and goiter. The infant may be small for gestational age. Occasionally, the infant will be exopthalmic. Onset usually occurs within the first week of life but may be delayed until the second week of life.

The immediate therapeutic concerns are cardiac failure and respiratory embarrassment secondary to goitrous encroachment on the trachea. Therapy must be instituted immediately and vigorously. Thionamide drugs (propylthiouracil (PTU) 10 mg/kg/day or methimazole 1 mg/kg/day in three divided doses) and iodides (SSKI, one drop three times a day) are utilized in all patients and should be maintained for 2-3 months. In the infant with severe tachycardia or cardiac arrhythmias, propranolol (3-5 mg/kg/day) should be utilized and digitalization may be necessary. If the neonate is extremely hyperactive, jittery, or irritable, phenobarbital (5 mg/kg/day) may be used in conjunction with propranolol and the standard drugs. If respiratory distress secondary to tracheal obstruction is suspected, lateral neck x-rays and blood gases must be obtained to evaluate the infant. All techniques to maintain airway and normal respiratory function must be utilized. If the obstruction is severe and respiratory collapse a real possibility, surgical intervention may be necessary. If surgery is necessary, subtotal thyroidectomy appears to be a safer procedure than tracheotomy.

Other less common complications including idiopathic thrombocytopenia purpura, infections and frontal bossing of the skull may occur. Long-term complications reported include premature closure of cranial sutures, advanced bone ages, ophthalmoplegias, and minimal cerebral dysfunction. Occasionally, neonatal Graves' disease may be more severe, persistent and resistant to treatment.[4]

ILLUSTRATIVE CASE

A 26-year-old primigravida white female during her second month of gestation developed a large soft goiter, exophthalmos, weight loss, and was diagnosed to be hyperthyroid. She was started on propylthiouracil (400 mg/day) and then maintained on 150 mg of propylthiouracil after she became euthyroid. At term, she delivered a 4 lb.-15 oz. male infant with normal apgar scores. The following day during routine neonatal examination, the infant was noted to have a large, soft goiter. The posterior fontanelle was closed and the anterior fontanelle was normal in size. The examination, including cardiovascular and lung findings were normal. T4, T3 and TSH levels were drawn. Lateral neck x-rays revealed a large anterior soft tissue mass encroaching upon the trachea. The mass did not cause any severe obstruction. The following day, the child was noted to be tremulous, had lost weight (4 lbs.-12 oz.), and had a pulse rate of 160. By late afternoon, the heart beat had increased to 200.

The infant was started on 20 mg propylthiouracil and 10 mg propranolol per day. The infant was also started on 1 drop of SSKI every 8 hours. Two hours after the second dose of propranolol, the infant was noted still to be extremely irritable and pulse rate was still 200. The propranolol was increased to 5 mg three times a day and phenobarbital 5 mg twice a day. The following morning, the infant was much less irritable, weight remained at 4 lbs.-12 oz., and pulse rate was 180. Medications continued unchanged for the next week with constant improvement demonstrated by decreasing pulse rate, and no evidence of tracheal obstruction. Weight gain remained slow. The results of the original thyroid function studies obtained on the second day of life revealed a T4 of 21.7 ug/%, T3 of 240 ng/% and a TSH of 2 μU/ml. The infant was discharged from the hospital at 14 days of age (weight 5 lbs.-4 oz.). At 24 days of age, he weighed 6 lbs.-1 oz. and was normal physically except for a persistent goiter. T4 was 8.3 ug/%. The propranolol was discontinued and the dose of propylthiouracil decreased to 5 mg every 8 hours. The SSKI was maintained at a drop every 8 hours. The child remained euthyroid and medication was discontinued at 3 months of age. The goiter was still palpable but smaller. By 5 months of age, the goiter was no longer present and the infant remained euthyroid.

CHILDHOOD GRAVES' DISEASE

Childhood hyperthyroidism is most often seen in adolescent females but may occur at any age in either sex. The most common presenting complaints in childhood are emotional lability (hyperactivity, restlessness, irritability or poor concentration), weight loss or goiter. Goiter is almost invariably found in children with Graves' disease.[5] Not infrequently this physical finding has not been noted by the parents or the patient. The most frequent findings in juvenile thyrotoxicosis, from the experience of one large children's medical center, is listed in Table VI.2. Exophthalmos is noted in slightly more than 50% of these children, but, fortunately, progressive exophthalmos and/or severe loss in visual acuity are rarely seen in childhood. Thyroid function tests will confirm the diagnosis since the normal range of values for thyroid function tests in childhood are very similar to normal adult values.

The treatment of Graves' disease in childhood is restricted because the use of radioactive iodine in children is controversial. Although radioactive iodine therapy has many proponents among internists, most pediatric endocrinologists do

TABLE VI. 2

MOST FREQUENT FINDINGS IN JUVENILE GRAVES' DISEASE*

SYMPTOM/SIGN	PERCENTAGE FOUND
Goiter	100
Tachycardia	65
Restlessness	60
Increased pulse pressure	57
Emotional lability	56
Proptosis	55
Thyroid bruit	44
Heat intolerance	41
Tremor	40
Polyphagia	40
Increased height	40
Diaphoretic	36
Fatigue	20

*Adapted from Vaidya et al.[6] with permission of the author.

do not recommend the use of radioactive iodine for treatment of juvenile thyrotoxicosis. It is well documented that the young (early infancy) thyroid gland is susceptible to tumor formation when exposed to radiation. Since it is not clear as to when or whether this suceptibility to the carcinogenic effects of radiation diminishes with age, there is concern about the possibility of a marked increase in thyroid carcinoma in these patients when they become 30 or 40 years of age. Furthermore, since the excretion of radioactive iodine is predominantly via the urinary tract, radiation of the prepubertal and adolescent gonads raises the spectre of future genetic malformations in the minds of pediatric endocrinologists.

The use of surgery as the treatment of choice for juvenile hyperthyroidism has strong proponents as well as strong opponents. The proponents of surgical treatment feel that this approach is not only the most expeditious but that the psychological effects of having a "chronic illness" engendered by the need for medication three times daily over a number of years is also avoided. However, the opponents of surgical treatment cite the high incidence of reoccurrence, the frequency of hypothyroidism and frequent occurrence of hypoparathyroidism and recurrent laryngeal nerve injury. In one study,[6] these latter two severe complications occurred once each in 33 children.

Medical therapy requires frequent and prolonged follow-up evaluation. The thioamide drugs must be taken approximately every 8 hours, an extremely difficult task for most adolescent and school aged children (especially the mid-afternoon dose). Relapses requiring further medical therapy or surgery occur in 50-60% of patients treated.[5] Toxic reactions (urticaria, serum sickness-like illnesses and agranulocytosis) occur in the range of 5 to 10%. The higher incidence of toxic reactions in children seem to be related to the higher dosages of thionamide drugs when calculated on a body weight basis. In a report by Amrhein and associates,[7] 10 patients of 38 children (26%) treated with PTU developed leukopenia and 7 patients had granulocytopenia. All but one of these patients were being maintained on dosages of PTU greater than 250 mg per day combined with thyroid hormone replacement therapy to prevent hypothyroidism.

Greer and associates[8] have suggested that short term medical therapy (until the patient becomes euthyroid) be utilized and surgery be performed if the patient relapses. This recommendation is based on their findings in adult patients that permanent remission is as likely to occur with short term as with long term therapy. The natural course of Graves' disease in childhood and adolescence differs from the experience of Greer and his associates. It has been documented in several large studies that approximately 35-50% of pediatric patients with Graves' disease have sustained remissions after 1-2 years of medical therapy.[5,9] With continued medical therapy, an additional small percentage of patients will sustain a remission. In the author's experience, approximately 60% of patients will have remission after 4-5 years of medical therapy.

It is clear that several therapeutic options are available. The following regimen is the author's own preference. Propylthiouracil (5-8 mg/kg/day or methimazole 0.5- 0.8 mg/kg/day) in three divided doses is used to initiate therapy. If cardiovascular symptoms are severe (marked tachycardia, flushing, severe heat intolerance or weakness) propranolol (2-5 mg/kg/day) is useful adjunctive therapy for the first 4-8 weeks. Complete blood count with differential counting of white cells is performed weekly during the first 6-8 weeks when high dosages of thioamide drugs are being utilized. Parents and the patients are of course warned to notify the physician of any unexplained fever, joint pains, urticaria, ecchymoses or petechiae, epistaxis or any other unusual symptom. The patient is monitored with thyroid function tests and the thioamide drugs reduced to dosages of 3-5 mg/kg/day for propylthiouracil and 0.3-0.5 mg/kg/day for methimazole. If the patient becomes hypothyroid on the lowest dosages of thioamide drugs (usually 100-150 mg of propylthiouracil or 10-15 mg of methimazole), L-thyroxine is added to prevent hypothyroidism. After 2 years, medication is discontinued and if the patient relapses, medical therapy is reinstituted for another 2 years. If the patient relapses once more, the therapeutic program then becomes more individualized and surgery is recommended. If the patient prefers to remain on medical therapy (and there has been no major difficulties with medical management), medical therapy can be reinstituted. If during the course of medical therapy, there are any major problems including poor compliance in terms of taking medication, any toxic reactions, medical therapy is discontinued and the patient prepared for surgery.

The preparation of a child with hyperthyroidism for thyroid surgery is similar to the preparations in adults. If possible, thioamide drugs should be utilized to suppress thyroid hyperfunction until the patient is euthyroid. Saturated solution of potassium iodide should be used in conjunction with thioamide drugs 2-3 weeks prior to surgery in order to reduce the vascularity and the size of the thyroid gland. Obviously, if the patient is hypersensitive to thioamide drugs, preparation using iodides alone will be necessary. Propranolol hydrochloride has been documented not to prevent operative thyroid crisis[10] but is certainly the drug of choice should thyroid crisis occur during or immediately after the operative procedure.

ILLUSTRATIVE CASE

L. M. presented at age 8 1/2 years because of fatigue and enlargement of the neck. Upon questioning, she admitted to diaphoresis, jitteriness, emotional lability and mild weight loss. She denied heat intolerance, diarrhea or weakness. Physically, she measured 134 cm and weighed 24 kg. She had mild exophthalmos, and some difficulty in convergence but no lid lag. She had a fine tremor on extension of her hands. The thyroid gland was three times normal size and there was a bruit. Her blood pressure was 120/60 and her pulse was 110. Her T4 was 14.4 ug% and her T3 resin uptake was 52% (both values being elevated).

She was treated with 250 mg of propylthiouracil for 8 weeks at which time her T4 was 6.0 μg%. The PTU was lowered to 150 mg/day and 3 months later decreased to 100 mg per day when her T4 was 5.2 μg%. She was maintained on this dose for 19 months. PTU then was discontinued. The goiter persisted throughout this time. She was seen 1 month after discontinuation of treatment and was found to be euthyroid clinically and biochemically. Less than one month later, she was noted to be losing weight (8 lbs.), restlessness in sleeping, and to have headaches, emotional lability, and palpitations of the heart. She was restarted on 300 mg of PTU and 30 mg of propranolol daily, and restored to euthyroidism in 6 weeks. Her dose of PTU was lowered to 150 mg per day. Her T4 after 6 months was $4.0 \mu g\%$ and therefore 0.1 mg of L-thyroxine was added to her therapeutic management. Two years later, when the patient was 12 years old, her PTU was discontinued. She was seen 4 weeks later and complained of palpitations. She had a blood pressure of 135/70 and a pulse of 120. She had no eye signs of Graves' disease. She did have a fine tremor of her extremities. Her thyroid gland was three times normal size. Her T4 was 12.6 ug%. Although surgery was recommended, the patient and parents elected to continue with medical therapy. PTU was reinstituted at 300 mg per day and then lowered to 200 mg and then 150 mg per day. After 2 years of further therapy, PTU was discontinued and no further relapses occurred.

REFERENCES

1. Fisher, DA: Laboratory diagnosis of thyroid disease. J Pediatr 82:1, 1973.

2. O'Halloran, MT and Webster, HL: Thyroid function assays in infants. J Pediatr 81:916, 1972.

3. Abvid J, Klein, AH, Foley, TP, et al.: Total and free tri-iodothyronine and thyroxine in early infancy. J Clin Endocr Metab 39:263, 1974.

4. Hollingsworth, DR and Mabry, CC: Congenital Graves' Disease. Am J Dis Child 130:148, 1976.

5. Vaidya, VA, Bongiovanni, AM, Parks, JS, et al.: Twenty-two years experience in the medical management of juvenile thyrotoxicosis. Pediatrics 54:565, 1974.

6. Bacon, GE and Lowry, GH: Experience with surgical treatment of hyperthyroidism in children. J Pediatr 67:1, 1965.

7. Amrhein, JA, Kenny, FM and Ross, D: Granulocytopenia, lupus-like syndrome and other complications of propylthiouracil therapy. J Pediatr 76:54, 1970.

8. Greer, MA, Kammer, H and Bouma, DJ: Short term antithyroid drug therapy for the thyrotoxicosis of Graves' disease. N Engl J Med 297:173, 1977.

9. Barnes, HV and Blizzard, RM: Antithyroid drug therapy for toxic diffuse goiter (Graves' disease): Thirty years experience in children and adolescents. J Pediatr 91:313, 1977.

10. Eriksson, M, Rubenfeld, S, Garber, AJ, et al.: Propranolol does not prevent thyroid storm. N Engl J Med 296:263, 1977.

CHAPTER VII

SPECIAL PROBLEMS IN THE TREATMENT OF HYPERTHYROIDISM

For a number of problems of hyperthyroidism it is best to consider treatment as a unit in terms of the specific problem rather than piecemeal in terms of specific modalities of therapy. The discussion will include hyperthyroidism in pregnancy, diseases which may produce symptoms of hyperthyroidism, and several of the more common complications of hyperthyroidism. In pregnancy it is necessary to consider the safety of the fetus and this will result in some modifications of the aims of therapy as well as the methods used to control the hyperthyroidism. When the symptoms of thyrotoxicosis occur in subacute thyroiditis, auto-immune thyroiditis, or choriocarcinoma, the aims of therapy must be tailored to the primary disease to produce improvement of these manifestations. Thus control of the primary disease controls the hyperthyroidism. A complication as thyroid storm, an acute exacerbation of the hyperthyroidism, demands a vigorous therapeutic program to insure survival of the patient. Treatment involves a combination of several agents to control the symptoms of these very toxic patients. A problem as thyrotoxic ophthalmopathy may proceed independently of the course of the other manifestations of hyperthyroidism. To save vision it may sometimes be necessary to add a glucocorticoid to diminish the severity of the ophthalmopathy or even to resort to surgery on the orbit.

HYPERTHYROIDISM IN PREGNANCY

The choices of therapy for the treatment of hyperthyroidism in pregnancy are quite limited. Radioiodine is absolutely contraindicated because of the radiation risks to the fetus. The use of any form of radiation in pregnancy always brings up the possibility of inducing some cellular damage in the fetus that may not appear until much later in the child. Furthermore, after twelve weeks gestation there is the important consideration of fetal thyroid ablation once the fetal thyroid begins to accumulate radioiodine. Special care must be taken to be sure that a patient is not pregnant before a radioactive isotope of iodine is used. When any doubt arises then a pregnancy test must be obtained to decide the issue. If inadvertant ^{131}I ablation has occurred in pregnancy, it is customary to allow the pregnancy to proceed to term.[1] Although the incidence of abortions and congenital anomalies differ little from normal pregnancies, there is little information about the long term effects on these offspring. Hypothyroidism and mental retardation occurred far more frequently in these children than might have been expected following uncomplicated pregnancies.

The selection of propranolol for use in pregnancy presents several problems. Certainly the drug permits effective control of the symptoms of hyperthyroidism and continued through pregnancy permits a choice of definitive therapy without need to consider the fetus. Unfortunately, the continued use of propranolol through pregnancy has been followed by small placenta, retarded fetal growth, fetal depression at birth, postnatal hypoglycemia and bradycardia.[2] Stimulation of uterine muscle plus direct fetal depression account for these problems. Propranolol should be used to control symptoms for a brief period, to prepare patients for surgery when the more conventional use of PTU and iodine is unsuitable and to treat thyroid storm. Propranolol however does not invariably prevent thyroid storm.[3]

In mild cases of hyperthyroidism it is tempting to allow the pregnancy to proceed without any treatment for the hyperthyroidism. Since it is usually the aim in controlling the symptoms of hyperthyroidism in pregnancy to allow a mild degree of hyperthyroidism to persist, it might be argued that mild, untreated hyperthyroidism will not interfere with the outcome of the pregnancy. Fetal safety would not be compromised by any of the drugs that might be employed in the treatment of hyperthyroidism. Unfortunately the incidence of premature delivery in uncontrolled hyperthyroidism is about 70%.[4] And as prematurity increases, infant survival decreases. It is therefore not wise to allow the hyperthyroidism to persist untreated.

With radioiodine eliminated as a choice and propranolol questioned in pregnancy therapy is either subtotal thyroidectomy or a course of a thioamide. The course after surgery is ordinarily quite satisfactory in the hands of experienced physicians and the infant survival compares quite favorably with that in uncomplicated pregnancies.[5,6] Even reservations about the safety of surgery in the first trimester of pregnancy are unwarranted since with recent experience the outcome remains the same irrespective of when the surgery is performed during prenancy.

Yet there are still some reservations about subtotal thyroidectomy in pregnancy. Hypothyroidism is not an infrequent complication of the procedure. Thus following subtotal thyroidectomy the outcome of the pregnancy improved in one group of patients when a thyroid supplement was added routinely following surgery.[7] This observation raises the suspicion that maternal hypothyroidism may well go unrecognized and endanger the survival of the fetus. Certainly there must be careful attention paid to the development of hypothyroidism following subtotal thyroidectomy in pregnancy. Hypocalcemia, though far less common than hypothyroidism, still is not unusual and fetal loss is alarmingly high in its presence.[8] Though hypocalcemia is not hard to recognize its correction may prove difficult and may persist for several weeks in spite of very aggressive therapy. Since preparation with a thioamide is necessary before surgery, the use of such drugs cannot be avoided even briefly during pregnancy. As the usual preoperative preparation with a thioamide requires from 6 weeks to 3 months to render a patient euthyroid, it will often be more advantageous to wait until after the pregnancy is completed before undertaking surgery. For the patient unwilling to continue the thioamide into the postpartum period surgery will be the only realistic choice regardless of the time that it might occur in pregnancy. The more rapid preparation with propranolol, which requires about 2 weeks and though successful in some hands,[9] is not entirely suitable for this purpose. As noted previously an adequate dose of propranolol may not always prevent thyroid storm. Propranolol must be continued intravenously postoperatively and then withdrawn slowly thereafter to avoid a recurrence of the symptoms of hyperthyroidism.

Special Problems in Treatment /103

In summary surgery requires adequate preoperative preparation, does not avoid the use of a thioamide, and introduces certain unavoidable complications.

There have been many objections to the use of thioamides in pregnancy. The thioamides easily cross the placental barrier[10,11] and may affect the fetal thyroid. Goiters have been observed in a small number of infants born to mothers who have received PTU during pregnancy.[12] There was no correlation with the dose of PTU or the maternal thyroid state. All of these goiters disappeared within three months after birth. It remains unclear whether PTU was the sole cause of the goiter or whether there was some predisposing condition such as the use of iodine, the presence of fetal hyperthyroidism at birth, or a subtle defect in thyroid hormone synthesis. With further observation it was clear that intelligence testing failed to demonstrate any difference from that of the offspring of normal pregnancies.[13]

Maternal hypothyroidism is easily recognized but the effects of a thioamide in this regard on the fetus are not always certain. It is not clear whether maternal and fetal thyroid states are always parallel. Since thyroid supplement can prevent maternal hypothyroidism its use in pregnancy has been suggested as a means of avoiding the effects of excessive doses of a thioamide on the fetus. The experience has been favorable when a thyroid supplement was added to PTU,[14,15] yet there is little evidence that thyroxine crosses the placenta in any appreciable degree.[16] It is much more satisfactory to carefully regulate the dose of PTU during pregnancy so as to avoid maternal hypothyroidism and only add a thyroid supplement if the maternal goiter enlarges.

The selection of PTU or MMI requires special thought in pregnancy. Of these two agents PTU is probably the better choice. Unfortunately the use of MMI in pregnancy has been followed by the occurrence of aplasia cutis in a small number of the infants.[17] PTU blocks the conversion of T4 to T3[18] and thus may aid in more rapid control of the maternal hyperthyroidism. If care is given to the control of the thyrotoxicosis with PTU then the potential of fetal hypothyroidism through this mechanism can be minimized.

The treatment of hyperthyroidism in pregnancy can be outlined as follows: Once the diagnosis of hyperthyroidism is established PTU is started at a dose of 100 mg every 8 hours. Should control be unsuccessful in one month the dose of PTU can be raised to 100 mg every 6 hours or if necessary to 200 mg every 6 hours. When euthyroidism is reached the dose of PTU can be reduced to maintain a level of thyroid function appropriate for pregnancy. Although the usual aim in hyperthyroidism is to render a patient fully euthyroid, this is probably not wise in the pregnant patient. A more satisfactory approach is to permit a mild degree of hyperthyroidism and to maintain the T4 in the normal range for pregnancy, a value just above the range of normal in the nonpregnant patient. If careful attention is paid to maintaining this degree of thyroid function, the outcome should be favorable to the fetus and to the mother as well. Following delivery the choice can then be made as to definitive therapy. The trial of PTU can be continued to a full year, the drug may be stopped as it would be in the short course of therapy, or surgery can be scheduled at a convenient time. For some patients the choice of definitive therapy may even be a dose of radioiodine. Figure 7.1 outlines the treatment of hyperthyroidism in pregnancy.

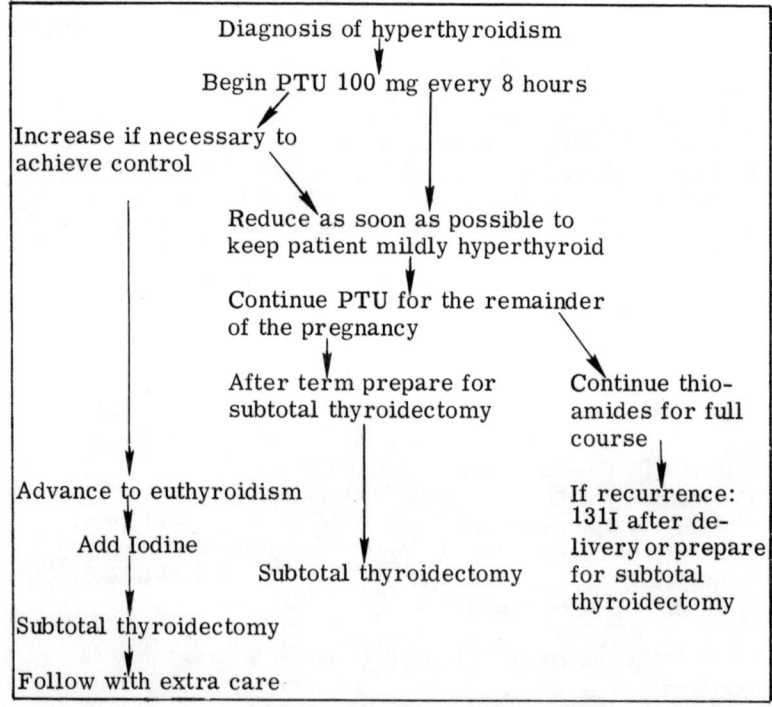

FIGURE 7.1: Treatment of hyperthyroidism in pregnancy

THYROID STORM

The successful treatment of thyroid storm requires both prompt diagnosis and vigorous therapy (Table VII.1). Mortality is high in the untreated patient and in fact when iodide was used as the sole means of therapy mortality was 60-70%.[19] An important step in the treatment of thyroid storm is to prevent its occurrence. It should be quite obvious that the reason for adequate preparation of the hyperthyroid patient for subtotal thyroidectomy with either a thioamide or propranolol is to prevent this catastrophy. Since many stresses may produce thyroid storm it is important to avoid elective surgery in the uncontrolled hyperthyroid patient and to recognize that storm can appear whenever another serious illness complicates thyrotoxicosis. Another important aspect of the treatment of thyroid storm is that diagnosis is usually based on clinical evidence alone. Thyroid function tests may actually be less elevated at the onset of storm than when the diagnosis of hyperthyroidism was first made.[19a] Signs as extreme restlessness, high fever, or tachycardia cannot always be used to differentiate thyroid storm from another illness complicating the course of the hyperthyroidism. Treatment should be started when the probability of storm is high rater than when there is absolutely no question about the certainty of the diagnosis.

The aims of therapy are to block the synthesis of the thyroid hormones, to prevent the release of the hormones from the thyroid, to prevent the peripheral effects of thyroid hormones, and to treat any concurrent illnesses. The choice of propranolol, iodides, thioamides, reserpine, and hydrocortisone will vary with the circumstances. Since the degree of toxicity is great and immediate control of the situation so important it is usually necessary to combine several of these agents rather than rely on just one. Considerations about definitive therapy must take second place behind the need for the most rapid response to therapy.

Propranolol and reserpine are used to control the severe manifestations of hyperthyroidism in thyroid storm. Guanethidine is not employed because of its delayed onset as well as the high incidence of postural hypotension with an effective dose of the drug. The rapidity with which propranolol produces its effect makes it an ideal agent in this circumstance.[20] Asthma and congestive heart failure (as in the less urgent situations) are contraindications to its use. In the obtunded patient it is possible to administer 1-2 mg every 4-6 hours using the slowing

TABLE VII.1
TREATMENT OF THYROID STORM

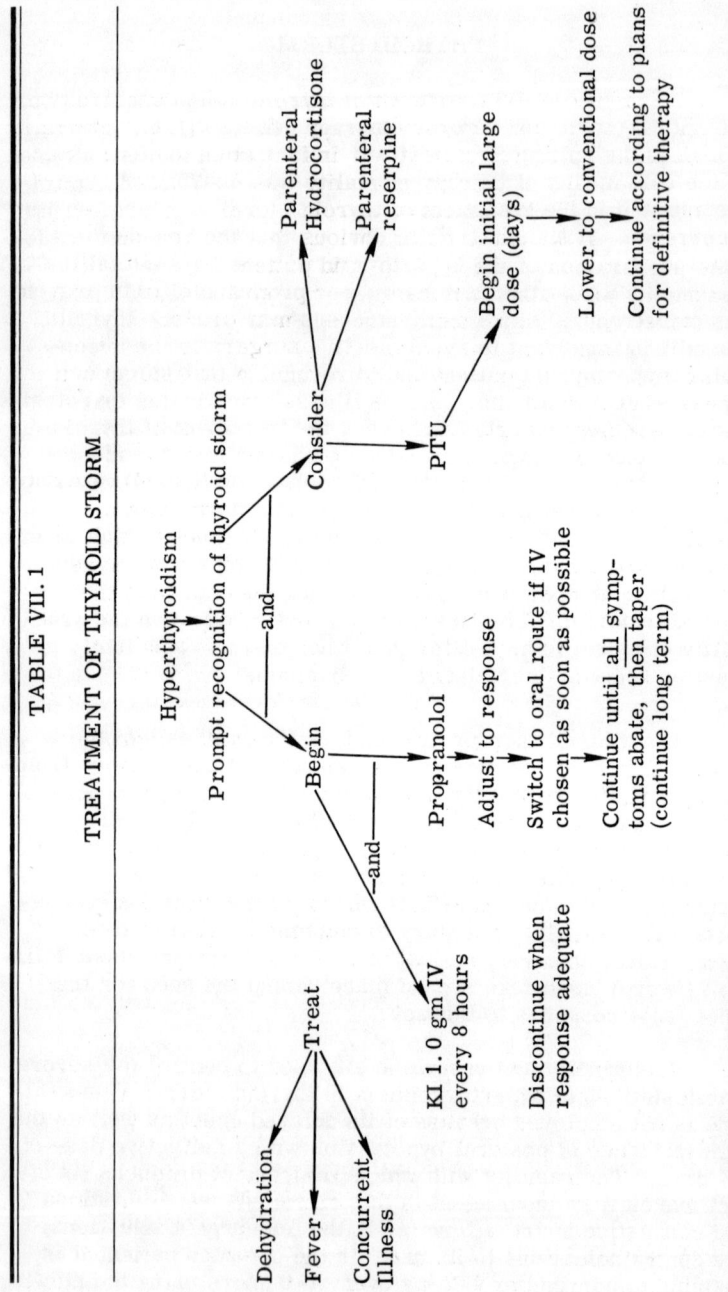

of the pulse rate as a guide. With an adequate dose the pulse will fall within a matter of several minutes, and when the pulse begins to return to the previous level the dose of propranolol should be repeated. Maximum benefit is usually achieved with the pulse rate at 100-110/minute. Once the patient can take oral medication 40-60 mg of propranolol can be substituted at 6-hour intervals. This dose of propranolol may also be used to begin therapy if the patient can take oral medication. The effect will be evident in a matter of hours so that the dose can be increased at 6-hour intervals as required until the pulse rate falls to 100-110/minute. It is wise to continue propranolol after full control of the hyperthyroidism has been achieved. Depending upon the future plans for therapy it can be tapered slowly over a several week period to avoid a flare in the symptoms.

Reserpine proved quite beneficial in controlling thyroid storm before propranolol was available.[21] At present the indications for reserpine are when sedation is required because of extreme agitation, when propranolol is contraindicated, or when the situation seems so urgent that a single agent will not suffice. The delay in response makes the oral preparation unsuitable for the treatment of storm. Reserpine should be administered intramuscularly beginning with 1 mg and then increasing the dose as required at 4-6 hour intervals until a response is achieved. The effect usually appears in about 8 hours and occurs with a dose of reserpine of 2-4 mg every 4-6 hours. As soon as the patient is stable the drug may be stopped.

In thyroid storm iodine is used to block the release of the stored hormones.[22] The benefit will occur within a matter of hours with either an oral or an intravenous preparation. Intravenously the dose is 1 gram of potassium iodide slowly over an 8-hour period. Orally the dose is 10 drops of Lugol's Solution every 8 hours. It is important to recall that in preparing the patient for subtotal thyroidectomy the dose of Lugol's Solution is only 2-3 drops three times daily. Iodides are continued for 3-4 days by which time maximum benefit from the drug should be apparent.

Although blocking the production of thyroid hormones would appear to be the most important step in the treatment of thyroid storm, there are a number of reasons why it proves unimportant. Since a parenteral form of a thioamide is not available, the medication can only be administered to the very ill patient in a crushed form through a nasogastric tube, a rather unsatisfactory route at best. Furthermore even when a thioamide can be started immediately, the benefit of blocking thyroidal hormone synthesis will not be evident until the pool of existing hormone diminishes through peripheral metabolism. The rapidity of the effects of thioamides will depend on the rate of turnover and will not appear for some time. The block by PTU in the conversion of T4 to T3[18] might have an additional benefit by lessening the effect of thyroid hormones on the cells immediately. There is an important reason for the addition of a thioamide to the regimen. Unless hormone production is blocked, the large amount of iodide customarily used to prevent the release of thyroid hormones will accumulate and can eventually supply enough iodide to raise the production of thyroid hormones either when escape from the block by iodides occurs or when the iodides are withdrawn.

The dose of PTU or MMI requires some qualification. To produce a complete block of thyroid hormone synthesis requires a dose of MMI[23] that has a high incidence of side effects.[24] Furthermore a full block with a thioamide may not be essential in any case.[25] For most situation 200 mg of PTU or 20 mg MMI every 6 hours will be sufficient. If circumstances make higher doses necessary then once control is achieved the dose of the thioamide should be reduced to these safer levels.

Additional therapeutic measures are in order. The patient must be kept well hydrated. Fever should be lowered with either alcohol sponges or a hypothermia blanket. For this purpose the use of aspirin must be used with care since salicylates have been shown to raise the levels of free T3 and T4.[25a] In the very urgent situations it is wise to administer 100 mg hydrocortisone every 8 hours intramuscularly. Adrenal insufficiency does not appear to be a significant factor in most cases of hyperthyroidism[26] but survival has improved in thyroid storm with the use of adrenal steroids.[19]

Several other approaches to the treatment of thyroid storm should be mentioned. When there is iodine hypersensitivity lithium may be considered. However the patient must be carefully monitored by the determination of plasma levels of lithium to maintain the dose of lithium within safe levels and avoid side effects.[27] In the very ill patients who have been resistant to other therapy plasmapheresis has been used successfully.[28]

The judicious combination of the usual drugs more often than not will control thyroid storm so that such heroic measures are rarely required.

The following case illustrates the treatment of thyroid storm. An 18-year-old woman was admitted to the hospital in June, 1977 for a subtotal thyroidectomy. The diagnosis of hyperthyroidism had been made about two years previously. In the two-year interval the thyrotoxicosis had been controlled first with MMI and then following an episode of serum sickness, PTU. One month before admission the appearance of a maculopapular eruption necessitated discontinuing the PTU. At the time of admission the patient complained of irritability, increased sweating, and weight loss. The thyroid was estimated at twice normal in size. The pulse was 140/minute at rest. A T4 was 17 mcg% (normal 5-12) and the T3 388 ng% (normal less than 190). The patient was prepared for surgery with propranolol and iodide. Within one week after admission at 60 mg propranolol every 6 hours her pulse was 90-100/minute at rest and 110/minute with exercise. She also received 3 drops of Lugol's Solution every 8 hours.

One day after surgery the patient became disoriented, agitated, and extremely restless. The propranolol had been continued after surgery as 1 mg intravenously every 6 hours. In addition to these symptoms her temperature was 102° rectally, and her pulse, 140/minute. As soon as the diagnosis of thyroid storm was made the dose of propranolol was adjusted to maintain the pulse below 100/minute and potassium iodide was started at 1 gram slowly every 8 hours. In the first 24 hours of therapy it was necessary to repeat the intravenous dose of propranolol every 4 hours. Because of the extreme agitation the patient was also started on reserpine 1 mg every 6 hours. Within 8 hours there was a marked improvement in the mental status of the patient. Her temperature had returned to normal, and her pulse had slowed to 100-110/minute. Over the second and third postoperative days the improvement continued and the patient was able to ambulate. On the third postoperative day the intravenous iodine, intramuscular reserpine, and intravenous propranolol were discontinued. Her only medication was propranolol (60 mg 6 hours orally). The remainder of her hospital stay was uneventful.

The case illustrates the fact that thyroid storm can occur despite adequate preparation with propranolol. It should be emphasized that the clinical details were kept brief to underscore the importance of the need to begin therapy of thyroid storm when suspicion is high. The dose of propranolol was adjusted to keep the pulse below 100. The combination of propranolol, iodine, and reserpine was chosen for several reasons. Iodine blocked the release of the thyroid hormones, propranolol,

some of the peripheral manifestations. In this case it was
necessary to add reserpine as well because of the extreme
agitation of the patient. Allergic reactions to PTU and MMI
prevented use of either thioamide. In spite of the marked degree of hyperthyroidism improvement occurred rapidly and
within two days of starting therapy for storm the patient was
ambulatory. As soon as her condition was stable, iodine and
reserpine were withdrawn. It was important to keep the duration of iodine therapy to a minimum since without a thioamide,
recirculation of iodide was not blocked and as noted before
another flare in the hyperthyroidism was possible. As an alternative to surgery ablation of the thyroid with ^{131}I would have
been far safer but the patient and her family had declined this
modality.

OPHTHALMOPATHY

Though the eye manifestations of Graves' Disease can
cause much concern in the management of the disease, these
resolve without therapy. The problems to consider are as follows: (1) How therapy of the hyperthyroidism influences the
progression of any eye problems; (2) Which complications will
require special therapy; and (3) What can be expected from the
available therapies for ophthalmopathy. Treatment often requires close cooperation between the physician managing the
hyperthyroidism and an ophthalmologist experienced in thyroid
eye disorders.

There are several facts to consider in the relationship
of the treatment of hyperthyroidism and the subsequent progression of eye problems. General observations about the
natural progression of these manifestations are pertinent.[29]
Exophthalmos when absent rarely appears after the hyperthyroidism is controlled. It usually reaches a peak early in the
course of the hyperthyroidism, and does not change during the
therapy. Spontaneous recovery is the rule in at least one-half of
the cases of ophthalmoplegia and lid retraction. There has been
much concern about the influence of surgery, radioiodine, or
thioamides in the progression of the ophthalmopathy. However,
there is little solid evidence favoring one method of treatment
or hyperthyroidism over another.[29,30] Even the fear that hypothyroidism accelerates exophthalmos remains unproven.[30]
Since specific therapy for eye problems often requires full control of the hyperthyroidism, it is probably most important to
achieve euthyroidism as rapidly as possible. If the progression
of the eye signs appears to parallel the control of the hyperthyroidism, then it is appropriate to alter the therapy of hyperthyroidism.

Special Problems in Treatment /111

Mild eye manifestations, outlined in Chapter I, usually require only local care. When lid retraction interferes with lid closure, it is necessary to protect the cornea from dust injury with protective glasses or an eye patch. Many time the severity of this problem will not be apparent until the patient is examined for lid closure when recumbent or questioned carefully. A 1/2% methyl cellulose solution, for example, will provide lubrication and relief for the annoying, gritty sensation that disturbs these patients. Minimal periorbital edema usually respond to diuretic therapy. All in all for patients with these Class II changes in the scheme proposed by Werner[21] reassurance of the patient is sufficient.

More severe forms of infiltrative ophthalmopathy can proceed with surprising rapidity to destroy vision and even result in loss of the involved eye. As protrusion of the eye advances chemosis becomes a significant source of disability. There is also the problem of secondary infection of the exposed and unprotected globe. Optic neuritis is probably a direct result of the damage produced by the increased orbital contents on the optic nerve.[32] The process which often involves the muscles of the orbit itself and which produces various forms of paralysis rarely requires immediate therapy in spite of the disabilities produced. The choices of therapy for these problems include the systematic use of corticosteroids, the administration of radiation to the orbit and pituitary, and finally surgical intervention.

didn't work for me

Of the three choices of therapy corticosteroids are the mainstay of therapy. The key to adequate therapy is to use a dose high enough and to begin it as early in the course of the ophthalmopathy as possible. The exact indications for beginning steroids are flexible but in general are those of steadily increasing proptosis over several weeks, severe chemosis, or optic neuritis. For most situations prednisone in a total daily dose of 40 mg will suffice and improvement will appear within the first week of therapy. As the problem stabilizes the prednisone may be reduced slowly over several weeks. The guide to the reduction is the stability of the eye problem. If the disease flares then the dose must be increased; if the disease remains stable then further reduction of the dose is possible. Occasionally it will be necessary to increase the dose of prednisone to 120-140 mg daily.[33] The average duration of therapy with prednisone varies from 6-12 months. Unfortunately even with 120-140 mg of prednisone some patients will not respond. Ophthalmoplegia rarely improves with corticosteroids.[34] It is essential that care be taken to avoid the adverse effects of large doses of steroids and this must be kept in mind whenever steroids are considered.

Many alternative medical approaches for progressive ophthalmopathy have appeared over the years. Retrobulbar injections of corticosteroids[35] offer an alternative to systemic steroids when the situation is less urgent. The response is not as satisfactory as with systemic steroids and the method of administration is often quite distressing to the patient. Guanethidine applied as eye drops has been suggested in milder cases,[36] but the response is not very impressive. The success with total thyroid ablation using radioiodine[37] was not confirmed by others.[38] Immunotherapy with azathiopurine has not influenced the course of infiltrative ophthalmopathy[39] and its routine use to prevent the progression of these manifestations has little to recommend it.[40] The beneficial effect of thyroxine supplements in reducing the progression of proptosis following radioiodine ablation for the hyperthyroidism remain unexplained[41] and unconvincing.

There have been several forms of radiation therapy used in the treatment of exophthalmos. Conventional irradiation has been directed to the pituitary as well as to the orbit. The mechanisms for the improvement with the latter remains obscure.

The improvement with conventional irradiation does not compare favorably with systemic corticosteroids and the improvement takes many months to appear. The risk of hypopituitarism is always a consideration with irradiation to the pituitary especially since the secondary adrenal insufficiency will necessitate constant, life long adrenal steroid replacement. Supravoltage irradiation is more promising.[43] Here again rapidly progressive exophthalmos is the primary indication. Depending on availability it may offer an alternative to corticosteroids and should be considered whenever surgery is contemplated on the orbit. The beneficial response to supravoltage irradiation does not correlate with immune factors such as the Long Acting Thyroid Stimulator or antithyroid antibodies. Ophthalmoplegia remains unchanged regardless of the effect on the exophthalmos.

Three surgical approaches, transantral, transfrontal, and lateral[44,45,46] have been used to decompress the orbital contents. The transantral and the transfrontal methods produce comparable benefits. However, the former leaves no visible incision and is a shorter procedure whereas the latter permits a more extensive exploration of the contents of the orbit.[47] Neither method is without risk. Diplopia often follows the transantral decompression.[48] Frontal lobe damage, central nervous system infection, cerbrospinal rhinorrhea, and global pulsation may follow the transfrontal decompression.[49] Furthermore a small number of patients will not benefit from orbital decompression. None of the surgical procedures consistently helps ophthalmoplegia. The indications for orbital decompression include the following: Deteriorating visual acuity, increasing constriction of the visual fields, or ulceration of the cornea. Considering the complications of surgery it is not easy to use cosmetic appearance as an indication for orbital decompression. Whether or not corticosteroids should always be used before considering surgery will depend on the rapidity with which the infiltrative changes occur, the dose of steroids that might be required, and the surgical expertise available.

Correction of ophthalmoplegia should follow control of the hyperthyroidism as improvement often occurs during therapy.[50] Surgery is indicated when paralysis of external ocular muscles produces diplopia or when ptosis produces significant cosmetic deformity. The sequence of surgical procedures is usually orbital decompression, correction of the opthalmoplegias causing the diplopias, and finally correction of the lid retraction. This sequence will yield the most satisfactory results with regard to both eye muscle function and appearance of the eyes. The decision about which eye muscles will require correction is often decided at surgery by means of forced function of all eye muscles. The impairment of function results from fibrosis and the subsequent adhesions between groups of muscle bundles so that surgical correction must often include recession of the inferior and medial muscles as well as separation of adhesions.[51] Preoperative examinations often fail to demonstrate the full extent of involvement of each group.

UNUSUAL FORMS OF HYPERTHYROIDISM

In many diseases symptoms of hyperthyroidism will arise and require therapy. Signs and symptoms of hyperthyroidism may occur in such primary thyroid disorders as subacute thyroiditis,[52] autoimmune thyroiditis,[53] painless thyroiditis,[54] or thyroid carcinoma.[55] A similar dilemma may arise during the course of such neoplasms as choriocarcinoma,[56] embryonal carcinoma of the testes,[57] struma ovarii,[58] or hydatidiform mole.[59] Hyperthyroidism may occur secondary to a pituitary or hypothalmic disorder.[60, 61] Finally hyperthyroidism may result from administration of exogenous hormone, or from an unwanted effect of exogenous iodides.[62, 63] This list includes many unrelated disorders, some common, others quite unusual. The unifying element is to recognize that therapy directed toward the primary disorder will usually produce an amelioration of the hyperthyroidism. Although in most of these settings the primary problem is quite obvious, sometimes the appearance of hyperthyroidism occurs first.

The association of hyperthyroidism with neoplasms is quite unusual and the course of the former improves with treatment of the latter. However severe hyperthyroidism may occur and symptomatic control of the hyperthyroidism will be required.[64] Clinical improvement has been achieved with iodine but since many of these reports antedate propranolol, the latter should be considered as well. As to prognosis only struma ovarii is favorable in outlook since the degree of malignancy is often low grade. Ablation with ^{131}I for this tumor should be considered since true thyroid tissue derived from the neoplasm produces the excess supply of thyroid hormones.[58, 64]

As a rule hyperthyroidism appears in the more severe forms of subacute thyroiditis. Rarely the thyroiditis may be painless and hyperthyroidism the only feature.[54] The process is self-limited and therapy must be directed toward the thyroiditis. Most patients respond within days to 40 mg of prednisone in divided doses. Once remission is achieved the dose can be reduced slowly over a period of several months. Thioamides are not appropriate since a damaged gland leaks thyroid hormones. When necessary propranolol can be added to produce rapid symptomatic relief.

Thyrotoxicosis may follow or even occur in the course of autoimmune thyroiditis.[53, 65] The differentiation of the latter from the usual form of hyperthyroidism may be quite difficult. As with subacute thyroiditis the importance is that treatment of the thyroiditis is the aim of therapy.[66] It should be noted the complications of recurrence of hyperthyroidism and the appearance of hypothyroidism have been attributed to this form of thyroiditis.

Hyperthyroidism may follow the use of iodides in nontoxic goiter,[67] the use of thyroid supplement for a variety of reasons,[68] or the use of iodine-containing x-ray contrast material.[62] The hyperthyroidism may persist after the offending source of iodine is withdrawn so that a definitive modality of therapy will be required. The choice of ^{131}I ablation, a course of a thioamide, or subtotal thyroidectomy will depend on the usual variables encountered in hyperthyroidism. It is important to recognize that spontaneous remission is probably no different than when iodine is not the reason for the hyperthyroidism.

Large doses of a thyroid supplement are usually well tolerated. Uncommonly a syndrome resembling thyroid storm may appear.[69] When severe, this form of hyperthyroidism can be treated with propranolol until the thyroid hormones are metabolized and the toxicity disappears.

APATHETIC HYPERTHYROIDISM

In some patients the manifestations of hyperthyroidism differ from the usual hyperkinetic symptoms and include those of depression, apathy, as well as such cardiovascular problems as congestive heart failure or atrial fibrillation.[69] It is important to recognize that although the mode of presentation may be unimpressive with regard to the severity of the hyperthyroidism the outcome without prompt therapy may be fatal. These patients though not hyperkinetic have not tolerated the thyrotoxicosis well. A key to therapy is that in evaluating such patients the index of suspicion must be high. Most are above forty years of age so that the definitive therapy will be ^{131}I ablation. Considering the fragile nature of the situation it is best whenever possible to initiate therapy with a thioamide to render the patient less toxic before administering the therapeutic dose of radioiodine. For most of these patients it will not be possible to use any agents as propranolol, reserpine, or guanethidine to control symptoms. If necessary one of the iodine preparations will serve to control symptoms. Cardiovascular manifestations must be treated in the conventional manner.

REFERENCES

1. Stoffer, SS, Hamburger, JI: Inadvertent ^{131}I therapy for hyperthyroidism in the first trimester of pregnancy. J Nucl Med 17:146, 1976.

2. Glandstone, R, Hardf, A, Gersony, J: Propranolol administration during pregnancy: Effects on the fetus. Pediatr 86:926, 1975.

3. Eriksson, M, Rubenfield, S, Garber, AJ, et al.: Propranolol does not prevent thyroid storm. N Engl J Med 296: 263, 1977.

4. Mestman, JH, Manning, PR, Hodgman, J: Hyperthyroidism and Pregnancy. Arch Intern Med 134:434, 1974.

5. Talbert, LM, Thomas, CG Jr, Holt, WA, et al.: Hyperthyroidism during pregnancy. Obstet Gynecol 36:779, 1970.

6. Hawe, P: The management of thyrotoxicosis during pregnancy. Br J Surg 52:731, 1960.

7. Bell, GO, Hall, J: Hyperthyroidism and pregnancy Med Clin N Amer 44:363, 1960.

8. Worley, RJ, Crosby, WM: Hyperthyroidism during pregnancy. Am J Obstet Gynecol 119:150, 1974.

9. Levy, CA, Waite, JH, Dickey, R: Thyrotoxicosis and pregnancy. Use of preoperative propranolol for thyroidectomy. Am J Surg 133:319, 1977.

10. Peterson, RR, Young, WC: The problem of placental permeability for thyrotropin, propylthiouracil and thyroxine in the guinea pig. Endocrinology 50:218, 1952.

11. Marchant, B, Brownlie, BEW, McKay, D, et al.: The placental transfer of propylthiouracil methimazale, and carbimozole. J Clin Endocrinol 45:1187, 1977.

12. Burrow, GN: Neonatal goiter after maternal propylthiouracil therapy. J Clin Endocrinol Metab 25:403, 1965.

13. Burrow, GN, Klatskin, EH, Genel, M: Intellectual development in children whose mothers received propylthiouracil during pregnancy. Yale J Biol Med 51:151, 1978.

14. Herbst, AL, Selenkow, HA: Hyperthyroidism during pregnancy. N Engl J Med 273:627, 1965.

15. Selenkow, HA: Antithyroid - thyroid therapy of thyrotoxicosis during pregnancy. Obstet Gynecol 40:117, 1972.

16. Fisher, DA, Lehman, H, Lackey, C: Placental Transport of thyroxine. J Clin Endocrinol Metab 24:393, 1964.

Special Problems in Treatment /117

17. Mujtaba, Q, Burrow, GN: Treatment of hyperthyroidism in pregnancy with propylthiouracil and methimazole. Obstet Gynecol 46:282, 1975.

18. Saberi, M, Sterling, FM, Utiger, RD: Reduction in extrathyroidal triiodothyronine production by propylthiouracil in man. J Clin Invest 55:218, 1975.

19. Waldstein, SS, Slodki, SJ, Kaganiec, I, et al.: A clinical study of thyroid storm. Ann Intern Med 52:626, 1960.

19a. Jacobs, HS, Mackie, DB, Eastman, CJ, et al.: Total and free triiodothyronine and thyroxine levels in thyroid storm and recurrent hyperthyroidism. Lancet 2:236, 1973.

20. DAS, G, Krieger, N: Treatment of thyrotoxic storm with intravenous administration of propranolol. Ann Intern Med 70:985, 1969.

21. Dillon, PT, Babe, J, Meloni, CR, et al.: Reserpine in thyrotoxic crisis. N Engl J Med 283:1020, 1970.

22. Wartofsky, L, Ransel, BJ, Ingbar, SJ: Inhibition by iodine of the release of thyroxine from the thyroid glands of patients with thyrotoxicosis. J Clin Invest 49:78, 1970.

23. Berson, SA, Yallow, RS: Quantitive aspects of iodine metabolism. J Clin Invest 33:1533, 1954.

24. Wiberg, JJ, Nuttall, RQ: Methiazole toxicity from high doses. Ann Intern Med 77:414, 1972.

25. Nakashima, T, Taurog, A, Riesco, G: Mechanism of the action of thioureylene antithyroid drug. Factors affecting intrathyroid metabolism of propylthiouracil and methimazole in rats. Endocrinology 103:2187, 1978.

25a. Larsen, PR: Salicylate - induced increase in free triiodothyronine in human serum. J Clin Invest 51:1125, 1972.

26. Giustina, G, Reschini, E, Valentini, F, et al.: Growth hormone and cortisol responses to insulin-induced hypoglycemia in thyrotoxicosis. J Clin Endocrinol Metab 32: 571, 1971.

27. Eulry, F, Orgiazzi, J, Mornex, R: Les sels de lithium ont-ils leur place dans le traitement des hyperthyroidis graves? Nouv Presse Med 6:2955, 1977.

28. Ashkar, FS, Katims, RB, Smoak, WM, et al.: Thyroid storm. Treatment with blood exchange and plasmapheresis. JAMA 214:1275, 1970.

29. Hales, IB, Rundle, FF: Ocular changes in Graves' disease. Quart J Med 113:113, 1960.

30. Hamilton, RD, Mayberry, WE, McConahey, WM, et al.: Ophthalmopathy of Graves' Disease: A comparison between patients treated surgically and patients treated with radioiodine. Clin Proc 42:812, 1967.

31. Werner, SC: Modification of the classification of the eye changes of Graves' disease: Recommendations of the ad hoc committee of the American Thyroid Association. J Clin Endocrino Metab 44:203, 1977.

32. Trobe, JD, Glaser, JS: Dysthyroid optic neuropathy. Arch Ophthamol 96:1199, 1978.

33. Werner, SC: Prednisone in the emergency treatment of malignant exophthalmos. Lancet 1:1004, 1966.

34. Brown, J, Coburn, JW, Wigod, RA, et al.: Adrenal steroid therapy of severe infiltrative ophthalmopathy of Graves' disease. Am J Med 34:786, 1963.

35. Thomas, ID, Hart, JK: Retrobulbar repository corticosteroid therapy in thyroid ophthalmopathy. Med J Aust 2:484, 1974.

36. Sneddon, JM, Turner, P: Adrenergic blockade and the eye signs of thyrotoxicosis. Lancet 2:525, 1966.

37. Bauer, FD, Catz, B: Radioactive iodine therapy for progressive malignant exophthalmos. Acta Endocrinol 51:15, 1966.

38. Boyle, IT, Greig, WR, Thomson, JA, et al.: Effect of thyroid ablation on dysthyroid exophthalmos. Proc Soc Med 62:19, 1969.

39. Burrow, GN, Mitchell, MS, Howard, RO, et al.: Immunosuppressive therapy for the eye changes of Graves' disease. J Clin Endocrinol Metab 31:307, 1970.

Special Problems in Treatment /119

40. Winand, RJ, Mahieu, P: Prevention of malignant exophthalmos after treatment of thyrotoxicosis. Lancet 1: 1196, 1973.

41. Koutras, DA, Alexander, WD, Buchanan, WW: Effect of thyroxine on exophthalmos in thyrotoxicosis. Br Med J 1:493, 1965.

42. Beierwaltes, WH: X-ray treatment of malignant exophthalmos. A report on 28 patients. J Clin Endocrinol Metab 13:1090, 1953.

43. Donaldson, SS, Bagshaw, MS, Kriss, JP: Supervoltage orbital radiotherapy for Graves' disease ophthalmopathy. J Clin Endocrinol Metab 37:276, 1973.

44. Long, JC, Ellis, GD: Temporal decompression of the orbit for thyroid exophthalmos. Amer J Ophthamol 62:1089, 1966.

45. Calcaterra, JC: Paranasal sinus decompression of the orbit in Graves' disease. Ophthalmic Surg 8:80, 1977.

46. Ogura, JH: Transantral orbital decompression for progressive exophthalmos: A follow up of 54 cases. Med Clin North Am 52:399, 1968.

47. Gorman, CA, Desanto, LW, MacCarty, CS, et al.: Optic neuropathy of Graves' disease. Treatment by transantral or transfrontal orbital decompression. N Engl J Med 290: 70, 1974.

48. Young, JDH: Ocular complications of transantral decompression for thyrotophic exophthalmos. Proc R Soc Med 64:929, 1971.

49. MacCarty, CS, Kenefick, TP, McConahey, WM, et al.: Ophthalmopathy of Graves' disease treated by removal of roof, lateral walls, and lateral sphenoid ridge. Review of 46 cases. Mayo Clin Proc 45:488, 1970.

50. Apers, RC, Bierlaagh, JJM: Indications and results of eye muscle surgery in thyroid ophthalmopathy. Ophthalmalogica 173:171, 1976.

51. Miller, JE, Von Heunen, W, Ward R: Surgical correction of hypotropias associated with thyroid dysfunction. Arch Ophthamol 74:205, 1965.

52. Greene, JM: Subacute thyroiditis. Am J Med 51:97, 1971.

53. Buchanan, WW, Alexander, WD, Crooks, J, et al.: Association of thyrotoxicosis and autoimmune thyroiditis. Br Med J 1:843, 1961.

54. Dorfmansg, Cooperman, MT, Nelson, R, et al.: Painless thyroiditis and transient hyperthyroidism without goiter. Ann Intern Med 86:24, 1977.

55. Federman, DD: Hyperthyroidism due to functioning metastatic carcinoma of the thyroid. Med 43:267, 1964.

56. Morley, JE, Jacobson, RJ, Melamed, J, et al.: Choriocarcinoma as a cause of thyrotoxicosis. Am J Med 60:1036, 1976.

57. Steigbigel, NH, Oppenheim, JJ, Fishman, LM, et al.: Metastatic embryonal carcinoma of the testes associated with elevated plasma TSH-like activity and hyperthyroidism. N Engl J Med 271:345, 1964.

58. Kempers, RD, Dockerty, MB, Hoffman, DL, et al.: Struma ovarii-Ascitic, hyperthyroid and asymptomatic syndrome. Ann Intern Med 72:883, 1970.

59. Higgins, HP, Hershman, JM, Kenimer, JG, et al.: The thyrotoxicosis of hydatidiform mole. Ann Intern Med 83:307, 1975.

60. Hamilton, CR, Adams, LC, Maloof, F: Hyperthyroidism due to thyrotopin-producing pituitary chromophobe adenoma. N Engl J Med 283:1077, 1970.

61. Emerson, CH, Utiger, RD: Hyperthyroidism and excessive thyrotropin secretion. N Engl J Med 287:328, 1972.

62. Blum, M, Weinberg, U, Shenkman, L, et al.: Hyperthyroidism after iodinated contrast medium. N Engl J Med 291:24, 1974.

63. Savoie, JC, Leger, FA, Massin, JP, et al.: L'hyperthyroidie induite par l'iode sur une glande thyroide apparemment normale. Nouv Press Med 5:2593, 1976.

64. Cave, WT, Dunn, JT: Choriocarcinoma with hyperthyroidism: Probable identity of the thyrotropin with human chorionic gonadotropin. Ann Intern Med 85:60, 1976.

65. Gavras, I, Thomson, JA: Late thyrotoxicosis complicating autoimmune thyroiditis. Acta Endocrinol 69:41, 1972.

66. Braverman, LE, Ingbar, SH, Vagenakis, AG, et al.: Enhanced susceptibility to iodide myxedema in patients with Hashimoto's disease. J Clin Endocrinol Metab 32:515, 1971.

67. Vagenakis, AG, Wang, C, Burger, A, et al.: Iodine-induced thyrotoxicosis in Boston. N Engl J Med 287:524, 1972.

68. Dymling, J, Becker, DV: Hyperthyroidism after thyroid hormone. J Clin Endocrinol Metab 27:1487, 1967.

69. Schottstaedt, ES, Smoller, M: 'Thyroid Storm' produced by acute thyroid hormone poisoning. Ann Intern Med 64:847, 1966.

70. Thomas, FB, Mazzaferri, EL, Skillman, TG: Apathetic thyrotoxicosis: A distinctive clinical and laboratory entity. Ann Intern Med 72:679, 1970.

INDEX

Agranulocytosis with
  thioamides, 30
Adrenergic-blocking agents,
  44-48

Carcinoma
  nonthyroid and hyper-
    thyroidism, 114
  nonthyroid after radioiodine
    therapy, 83
  struma ovarii, 10, 113
  of thyroid in hyperthyroid-
    ism, 10, 59
  of thyroid after radio-
    iodine therapy, 83-84
Corticosteroid therapy
  in ophthalmopathy, 111
  in thyroid storm, 108
  in thyroiditis and hyper-
    thyroidism, 114

Goiter, toxic adenomatous,
  6, 76
Guanethidine, 44

Hyperthyroidism
  apathetic, 15, 115
  atypical manifestations, 4
  in childhood, 94-97
  in childhood, case study,
    97
  clinical index, 3-4
  euthyroid (Graves'), 8
  neonatal, 91-93
  neonatal, case study, 93
  recurrence after subtotal
    thyroidectomy, 54
  T3, 10
  thyrotropin in, elevated,
    11

Hypocalcemia
  after subtotal thyroid-
    ectomy, 56
  after subtotal thyroid-
    ectomy, case study,
Hypothyroidism
  after radioiodine therapy,
    82
  after radioiodine therapy,
    case study, 82-83
  after subtotal thyroid-
    ectomy, 54-56

Iodides and Iodine
  in hyperthyroidism, 48-49
  hyperthyroidism following
    use of, 114-115
  in preparation for subtotal
    thyroidectomy, 59-60
  in thyroid storm, 107

Lithium, 49, 108

Ophthalmopathy
  corticosteroids in, 111
  infiltrative, 5
  irradiation for, 112
  natural course, 110
  noninfiltrative, 5
  orbital surgery for, 112-113

Perchlorate, as antithyroid
  drug, 24
Pregnancy
  and hyperthyroidism, 101-104
  flow diagram of hyperthyroid
    therapy, 104
Propranolol
  in hyperthyroidism, 46-48
  in pregnancy, 101

in thyroid storm, 106-107

Radioiodine therapy
 in children, 75
 dose selection, 78-81
 flow diagram of use in
  hyperthyroidism, 86
 mechanism of action, 73-74
 patient selection, 74-78
 in pregnancy, case study,
  74
 or thioamide, case study,
  77
 use of isotope ^{125}I, 73
Radioiodine uptake (RAI in
 hyperthyroidism, 14
Reserpine
 in hyperthyroidism, 46
 in thyroid storm, 107

Subtotal thyroidectomy
 in childhood, 95-97
 in childhood, case study,
  97
 and hypothyroidism, 54-57
 nerve damage in, 56
 in pregnancy, 102
 preparation of patients
  for procedure, 59-64
 propranolol preparation,
  case study, 62
 and recurrence of hyper-
  thyroidism, 54-57
 selection of patients,
  58-59
 surgical techniques, 67-71
 thioamide preparation,
  case study, 62-64
 therapy flow diagram, 61

Thioamides (Thionamides):
 chemical structure, 24
 in childhood, 96-98
 complications of therapy,
  30-33
 as definitive therapy, 25-28
 failure of response, case
  study, 35-38

 mechanisms, 28-30
 in pregnancy, 103-104
 remission with therapy,
  case study, 37
 therapy flow diagram, 38
 toxicity, case study, 32
Thyroid function tests in
 hyperthyroidism:
 free thyroxine index, 10
 perchlorate washout test for
  thioamide response, 36
 T3 determination, 14
 T4 determination, 12
Thyroiditis:
 Hashimoto's Disease and
  hyperthyroidism, 10
 subacute and hyperthyroidism, 10
 therapy of hyperthyroidism
  in, 114
Thyrotoxicosis factitia, 8, 115
Thyroid storm, 105-110
Thyrotropin releasing factor,
 test in hyperthyroidism (TRH
 Test), 15
Thyrotropin (TSH) and suppression in hyperthyroidism, 11